NEONATAL AND PERINATAL SCREENING: THE ASIAN PACIFIC PERSPECTIVES

Neonatal and Perinatal Screening: The Asian Pacific Perspectives

Proceedings of the Second Asian Pacific Regional Meeting of the International Society for Neonatal Screening, Hong Kong, 28 November to 1 December 1995

Edited by

Stephen TS Lam, MD, FRCP

Head, Clinical Genetic Service,
Department of Health, Hong Kong

Calvin CP Pang, BSc, DPhil

Professor, Department of Chemical Pathology
The Chinese University of Hong Kong

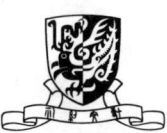

The Chinese University of Hong Kong

ISBN 962–201–765–7

THE CHINESE UNIVERSITY PRESS
The Chinese University of Hong Kong
SHA TIN, N. T., HONG KONG
Fax: (852) 2603 6692
E-mail: cup@cuhk.edu.hk
Web-site: http://www.cuhk.edu.hk/cupress/w1.htm

Printed in Hong Kong

Contents

The Second Asian Pacific Regional Meeting of the International Society for Neonatal Screening, Hong Kong, 28 November to 1 December 1995

Patron
SH Lee

International Advisers
Rui-Guan Chen (China)
Kwang-Jen Hsiao (Taiwan)
Ichiro Matsuda (Japan)
Hiroshi Naruse (Japan)
Bent Norgaard-Pederson (Denmark)
Brad L Therrell (USA)
Dianne R Webster (New Zealand)
Veronica Wiley (Australia)

Organizing Committee
Stephen TS Lam (Chairman)
Mike KM Tsui (Secretary)
Veronica MS Lam (Treasurer)
Calvin CP Pang (Scientific Programme)
WK Chan (Venue & Accommodation)
Belinda FH Leung (Social Functions)
Eric LK Law (Exhibition & Sponsorship)
Anita YY Ng (Publicity & Publication)

Preface

The need for screening for inherited metabolic diseases and endocrinopathies have been receiving attention and approval from medical workers and authorities in different parts of the world over the last 30 years. A series of international neonatal screening symposia has been conducted since 1966 to facilitate exchange of ideas and experiences. International liaison was further consolidated in the form of the International Society for Neonatal Screening (ISNS), which was inaugurated in 1991. The publication of the journal SCREENING in 1992 by this society was another significant landmark in the history of neonatal screening. To facilitate discussion at the regional level, it had been suggested in the first ISNS general meeting that regional meetings should be organized. Subsequently, the first such meeting in Asia was organized in Sapporo, Japan, in 1993.

During a business discussion of the first Asian Pacific Regional Meeting (APRM) of the ISNS, 1993, it was proposed that the second APRM should be conducted in Hong Kong. As the only delegate from Hong Kong, one of us (S.L.) was immediately put on the spot. Two issues were brought up. First, when the idea of having an APRM was initiated some years ago, the first meeting was originally planned to be held in Shanghai in 1990. For various reasons, the plan could not materialize. It would seem logical, however, for the second APRM to be conducted in Shanghai. Second, should the second meeting be held in Hong Kong, the most appropriate organization to host it would be the Hong Kong Society of Medical Genetics (HKSMG). However, up till then, this society did not have the experience of conducting such a big international event. It was only after a couple of months that the final decision was made — the HKSMG was bestowed the honour of hosting this meeting. The lesson to learn during that exercise is that, don't attend a business meeting unless you are prepared.

In line with the goals of conducting a regional meeting, we set the theme for the second APRM as 'Screening for Congenital Diseases in the Asian Pacific Region'. As suggested by Professor H Naruse during the first APRM, we decided to include more topics of regional interest in the second APRM. Of the ten symposia in the meeting, four were dedicated to issues that were considered highly significant, for their prevalence and health impact, namely, hypothyroidism, glucose-6-phosphate dehydrogenase deficiency, thalassemia and congenital infections. We had not, however, neglected the classical models of screening for inherited metabolic disease. Two whole symposia were devoted to studying the new technologies in the investigation of congenital diseases. As mentioned earlier, technologies must be met with proper organization for effective screening. Two symposia were hence included to cover issues of management, standardization, quality assurance, programme evaluation and logistics, legalities and ethics. Since we believed that neonatal screening should not be separated from efforts in perinatal or prenatal screening, which essentially screened for the same groups of disorders, namely, congenital or inherited diseases, we included a number of presentation for prenatal screening for single gene disorders and chromosome diseases. From the quantity of presentations and the quality of the discussions in the meeting, and the publication of this proceeding, we are happy that our primary objectives for conducting this event were accomplished.

We are most grateful to the 220 participants who turned up from twenty countries and regions, mostly from the Asian Pacific area. We wish sincerely that most have brought home results of exchanges that would be useful to their own research and practices. We are particularly indebted to the international and local advisers for their significant input into organizing this meeting. Our thanks are also due to the Patron of the HKSMG, Professor SH Lee, and the director of Department of Health, Dr. Margaret Chan, who had been most generous in supporting and encouraging us throughout the whole period of organizing this meeting. We greatly appreciate the devotion and excellent work of members of the Organizing Committee and of the various sub-committees. It was their competence and effectiveness that contributed to the success of the Meeting.

Stephen TS Lam, MD, FRCP
Calvin CP Pang, BSc, DPhil

Perspectives

History of Neonatal Screening and Issues Specific to the Asian Region — To the Memory of Robert Guthrie

Hiroshi Naruse

Tokyo Institute of Medical Science and Department of Pediatrics, Kyorin University, Tokyo, Japan.

Abstract   *Neonatal screening was initiated by Robert Guthrie who passed away on June 24, 1995 at his daughter's home in Seattle, WA, USA. He always tried to help people who wanted to develop regional screening, even in the Asian Pacific area. During the late Sixties and the Seventies, he visited New Zealand, Australia and Japan to work with local people for the establishment of neonatal screening programmes. He seriously hoped to develop such programmes in Asia and the Middle East. This great wish should be taken up by his students in the Asian Pacific Area. We should also try to develop close international cooperation. This area has wide occurrence of iodine deficiency. I think that hypothyroid screening will be one of the most effective means to treat all endemic cretinism including mildly affected patients. I have learnt the necessity of "quality control system in neonatal screening" from Guthrie too. For us, the most important aim of a screening programme is the detection of the very mild form of disease in affected patients.*

Memory of Robert Guthrie

Robert Guthrie who was a real pioneer of a field of neonatal screening passed away on June 24, 1995 in Oregon, USA. He always tried to cooperate with those who really wish to establish a system of neonatal screening in various countries. He helped development of a nationwide screening in New Zealand and Japan and tried to cooperate with specialists in China, Taiwan and some other countries in Asia region. When I discussed with him about neonatal screening in different places in the world, he always wanted to know about recent development of the screening in

Table 1 Professional Career of R. Guthrie

Graduated from University of Minnesota	MD 1945, PhD 1946
National Institute of Health	1946–1949
Professor & Chairman, Department of Bacteriology & Immunology, University of Kansas	1949–1950
Assistant, Department of Chemotherapy, Sloan-Kettering Institute, Rye, NY	1951–1954
Principal Cancer Research Scientist, Rosewood Park Memorial Buffalo, NY	1954-1958
Research Associate Professor of Pediatrics, State University of New York at Buffalo (SUNYAB)	1958–1971
Professor of Microbiology, SUNYAB	1970–1974
Research Professor of Pediatrics, SUNYAB	1971–1974
Professor Emeritus of Pediatrics and Microbiology, SUNYAB	1985–1995

that place. With deep mourning and cordial thanks for him, I introduce his achievement in our field.

He contributed an important paper concerning an early history of Guthrie-screening method in the first issue of Journal SCREENING[1]. Often he mentioned that his BIA method should be replaced by more modern methods but the method is still used in many countries. A method using a filter paper could be applied not only to the neonatal screening but to population based screening in various ages. This method for blood collection is a very important tool in public health and will be getting much more importance in the future.

I think many people know that he wanted to defect even very mild form of the disorders which could be harmful for human development. Of course, he had understood a discussion from the cost-benefit point of view but he was saying that when we had very valuable blood samples from human babies, we should utilize them as much as possible. As a active member of the Parents Association of Handicapped, he knew a life with any disorders, even it was mild, could not be as happy as healthy individuals and we should try hard to prevent even such mild disorders. He often discussed the necessity to set up a cut off level as low as possible to eliminate the possibility of false negative cases.

He was also interested in quality control in screening programmes. He was the first person to start a kind of quality control survey in the neonatal screening. However, he had recognized that his way to send "standards" to his collaborative laboratories was not enough as a method for the quality control system. Therefore, when he knew that we were trying to establish a national quality control system for my country, he could suggest to me many important idea regarding the quality control system.

Quality Control in Neonatal Screening

When we discuss about quality control in neonatal screening, we should consider what is the most unique feature of the neonatal screening tests. The task of main technicians in neonatal screening laboratories are different from that in conventional service laboratory of clinical chemistry. The main technicians must pick up a few abnormal samples from many normal samples correctly. When they find a sample which should be dealt with as an abnormal one, they must start the proper action for making diagnosis as early as possible. They have to pick up even mild abnormal one in order to avoid a false negative case. For this purpose, they have to understand the meaning of the cut off levels in each screening test very well.

They have to do *important judgment* in everyday works very often. The quality control system in neonatal screening should be useful for such the important judgment. When I started our system of the quality control, I sent slightly abnormal samples with normal samples and asked technicians to pick up abnormal samples exactly. The system I introduced was quite different from that in usual clinical chemistry. After I started this system, technical people and specialists of the target diseases discussed what were proper cut off levels in various screening very often. In Japan, many people did various kind of good works regarding the cut off levels and this facts is one of the important results of QC system.

Cut-off Levels of TSH Screening

In this report, I concentrate mainly the cut off level of thyroid stimulating hormone (TSH) screening. We have many reports which describe missed cases of congenital hypothroidism (CH) patients who had very mild elevation of TSH in the 1st sample for the screening. Recently, S. Harada et al.[2] showed that they found many CH patients who showed late increase of TSH levels. In Japan, most screening laboratories had CH patients who showed TSH levels between 10 to 15µU/ml of whole blood. Besides, as a clinical psychiatrist, I have seen a few cases who had mild mental retarded condition or autistic condition and had mild elevation of TSH. I think these were suffering from mild CH but did not detect early enough.

When we missed a mild cases of CH patients through the newborn screening, the babies might have very mild dysfunction of the brain and might not be recognized for a long time and some of them might be never diagnosed during all their lives. It is often said in some countries that people never missed CH patients even using a rather high cut-off level of TSH. They have to do a very detailed survey bases on close cooperation with psychiatrists in their countries before they had such a confidence. I cannot understand why they can say so when we consider such a mild form of CH patients.

Thus, I would like to propose to set the cut-off level of TSH to be at 10 μU/ml lower. People may be afraid that such a cut-off level may cause very serious hazards regarding a large number of second samples request or referring to clinicians. However, results of TSH screening in Japan have shown that the rate of a second sample request is not so high when we ask doctors to avoid using iodine containing antiseptics. According to data of the QC system in Japan, good laboratories which do not have iodine containing antiseptics, the rate of the second sample request is around 0.5 ~ 0.8%.

Development of Neonatal Screening in East Asia

In Asia, many countries have serious problems of iodine deficiency (IDD). As a result of the effort of workers and governments in these areas, the number of obvious endemic cretinism is decreasing dramatically. In April 1995, B. Therrell, JL Dhondt, B. Wilcken and myself were invited to Thailand and had learnt about significant progress in this country. We were informed that the number of endemic cretinism dropped dramatically. However, W. Charoensiriwatana et al. did a pilot screening in IDD areas and the results of the pilot study showed that still there existed significant number of High TSH babies in that area. They suggested that TSH screening with anti-IDD measures should be useful to detect mild cases of iodine deficiency. In this case, I would like to emphasize the importance of low cut off level of TSH in such screening.

We are living in East Asia where there is a large population and a serious IDD problem. Though many countries in the area are developing rapidly, still General Domestic Products per Capita is rather low in comparing with industrialized countries. However, when we decided to start a nationwide screening in Japan many years ago, GDP/p of Japan was only around US$800. Considering the seriousness of the IDD problem and the general conditions in many countries in East Asia, I would like to emphasize that we should aim to develop neonatal screening for congenital hypothroid in East Asia as soon as possible. For this purpose, we should develop international cooperation in this area rapidly.

Recently, I was visited by a professor in Indonesia who was hoping to establish a nationwide screening in Indonesia and to produce ELISA kit for TSH in Indonesia. We will start cooperation between Indonesia and Japan. As the first step of the cooperation, I recommended her to try to send her co-workers to a training course titled "Technology in Neonatal Screening" which is organized by Japan International Cooperation Agency every year in Sapporo. The JICA training course provides training on how to make ELISA reagents.

Apart from the JICA training course there are many other training courses or other activities which are useful for the future development of neonatal screening in East Asia. However, I am afraid that people who need such information do not have access to such information very often. In order to stimulate development of neonatal screening in East Asia, we need to accelerate the process of international cooperation.

For this purpose, I would like to propose to establish an Asian Branch of International Society of Neonatal Screening. The main purpose of the branch at present will be exchange of necessary information based on proper communication system. I hope the branch will be useful for the development of neonatal screening in East Asia.

References

1. Guthrie R. The origin of newborn screening. Screening 1992;1:5–15.
2. Harada S., Ichihara N., Arai J., et al. Later manifestation of congenital hypothyroidism predicted by slightly elevated thyrotropin levels in neonatal screening. Screening 1995;3:181–92.

Newborn Screening: Reviewing the Past, Exploring the Future

Bradford L Therrell

Texas Department of Health, Austin, Texas 78759, USA.

Abstract *Newborn screening began with the work of Guthrie in the early 1960s. By the end of the decade, PKU newborn screening was present throughout the United States, Canada, Europe, Australasia and Japan. Automation of the mechanics of testing, along with commercial development of sensitive assays to detect congenital hypothyroidism, provided the impetus for expanded screening throughout the 1970s and 1980s. Today, screening in developed countries included advanced micro-techniques for a number of the analytes, computerized tracking systems, remote demographic data entry, and voice response systems. Screening results are confirmed through DNA techniques and it is likely that such techniques will be automated for screening use in the near future. New advances are also proceeding in mass spectrometry. On the other hand, developing nations continue to experience major financial, educational, and logistical problems in implementing screening programmes. Nationally, debt and population usually cause implementation problems. Developing programmes are often fragmented and disconnected small programmes exist which may unaware of other programmes within the country. In many cases, screening disorders are included for personal or political reasons rather than for public health reasons. Established and developing screening programmes continue to expand both the benefits and expectations of newborn screening. We must continue to provide international cooperation between developed and developing programmes in order to facilitate improvements in both quality and quantity of newborn screening. Japan has taken a lead role in providing laboratory training to nations seeking assistance. The US is working towards national standards in number of areas. WHO is providing limited support in some developing areas. We must continue to support international efforts to further all aspects of screening in order to provide improved health and outcome for all children.*

Historical Review

To those of us currently involved in newborn screening, it is sometimes difficult to realize that the first newborn screening programme using dried blood on filter paper only began in the early 1960s. Even though Garrod[1] first used the terminology "inborn errors of metabolism" in 1902, it was about 30 years before Folig[1] developed his diaper screening test for phenylalanine (PKU) in 1933, and another 20 years before Bickel[3,4] described successful dietary intervention for this inborn error. As is often the case, the long tedious processes that lead to discovery and treatment of a devastating condition are finally met with accelerated studies of detection procedures. As technology and science advance, all of these processes are made quicker and simpler. In the case of PKU, it was another 10 years after treatment was reported before Guthrie reported his filter paper screening test for PKU[5]. This was followed by reports of a number of other disorders detectable by similar testing protocols[6,7]. Testing filter paper samples from newborns for PKU spread quickly as a popular preventive health programme and the first international meeting to discuss the testing process was held in Dubrovnik, Yugoslavia in 1966.

As other researchers learned of the techniques with filter paper samples, their scientific curiosity and research abilities expanded the concept of newborn screening to disorders of higher prevalence in diverse population groups. Among these were included in Garrick's development of procedures for sickle cell disease testing[8], Dussault's procedures for detecting congenital hypothyroidism[9,10], and Pang's method for detecting congenital adrenal hyperplasia[12]. While the technical aspects of testing blood spots on filter paper were improving method sensitivities and specificity, the invention of an automated quadratic punching device by inventor Robert Phillips[6] opened the way to reduced labor costs for the tedious processes associated with sample preparation. Commercialization of the varied testing methods coupled with automated sample preparation led to even broader acceptance of the cost effectiveness and social benefits of newborn screening. This is turn made more credible the idea of government financial support.

Expansion of newborn screening from metabolic testing to include testing for hypothyroidism (with an increased incidence over PKU of about 5:1) led to a joint international meeting on both topics in Japan in 1981[13]. It was becoming apparent that international cooperation would be enhanced by development of international standards and so the next international meeting [which continued the idea of newborn screening (as opposed to metabolic screening)] expanded discussion into the area of programme and laboratory quality control[14]. An international meeting on quality assurance was held the next year and this meeting led to the formation of an International Society for Neonatal Screening (ISNS) in 1987. The first ISNS meeting was held in Sydney, Australia in 1990[15], and the first regional meeting of the Society occurred with the Asian-Pacific Regional meeting in Sapporo, Japan in 1993[16]. There has now been a second meeting of ISNS[17] and the meeting which we are now attending is the second Asian-Pacific Regional Meeting.

In the United States (U.S.) where screening first began, there is still no nationally mandated programme. Instead there are 53 separate programmes (including 50 states, the District of Columbia, Puerto Rico, and the Virgin Islands), each with its own regulations and each with a different set of screening disorders. Table 1 gives a summation of the disorders included in screening and the number of programmes that screen[18]. Despite a national mandate to screen entire programme populations for sickle hemoglobinopathies, there remain 6 programmes that maintain targeted (or voluntary) testing for this class of disorders.

A significant number of national efforts to improve and standardize newborn screening in the U.S. are currently in progress. The Council of Regional Networks for Genetic Services (CORN) has recognized the importance of newborn screening through its formation of a Newborn Screening Committee. Significant contributions to date include U.S. Newborn Screening Guidelines[19], Guidelines for Retention, Storage, and Use of

Table 1   Disorders Included in U.S. Screening Programs

Screening Disorder	Number of Programs	Percentage of Programs
Phenylketonuria	51	100
Hypothyroidism	51	100
Galactosemia	46	90
Sickle Cell Disease[a]	43	84
Maple Syrup Urine Disease	22	43
Biotinidase	19	37
Homocystinuria	17	33
Congenital Adrenal Hyperplasia	15	29
Cystic Fibrosis	3	< 1
Toxoplasmosis	2	< 1

[a] Include 6 programs with targeted testing.

Residual Blood Samples After Newborn Screening Analysis[20], and a
response to the Institute of Medicine Statement on genetic risks[21]. Addi-
tionally, CORN has sponsored symposia on issues and implications of
sickle cell screening[22], the impact of early hospital discharge on newborn
screening[23], and developing public health guidelines for genetic services
(including newborn screening[24]. The Association of State and Territorial
Public Health Laboratory Directors (ASTPHLD) sponsors symposia on
newborn screening at approximately 18 month intervals and has undertaken
a joint effort with CORN to develop a number of standards relating to
various aspects of the newborn screening system including nomenclature,
laboratory proficiency, submitter procedures, data management and other[25].
These two groups also cooperate to collect national data on newborn
screening for compilation into annual reports. The U.S. Department of
Health and Human Services has funded a consultation review team through
the Bureau of Maternal and Child Health whose expertise in medicine,
laboratory, quality assurance, and programme administration has now been
shared with over 15 programmes since 1987[26]. The National Committee for
Clinical Laboratory Standards (NCCLS) has been involved in newborn
screening through its publication of a national standard for blood collection
in filter paper and an accompanying videotape[27]. The American Academy
of Pediatrics has also taken a proactive approach to newborn screening. In
addition to various guidelines about metabolic and thyroid screening[28,29],
they have also published fact sheets[30,31] and goals for practicing
pediatricians[32].

The laboratory aspect of newborn screening is actively supported by
the Centers for Disease Control and Prevention (CDC) through its Infant
Screening Quality Assurance programme (ISQAP). In addition to quarterly
proficiency testing samples for a number of screening analytes, the CDC
also provides blood spot materials for quality control and calibration, and
provides education reports on each new production lot of commercial filter
paper approved for use in the U.S. Their services are also used by a large
number of laboratories outside of the U.S. All of these efforts are combin-
ing to improve the efficiency, and effectiveness of a newborn screening
system that is national in scope but regional in its administration.

Developing Countries

Newborn screening continues to expand around the globe. Each year
more developing countries include newborn screening in their public health

priorities. In 1993, Velazquez reviewed 35 programmes in 21 developed countries[33]. Surprisingly, he found that there were over a dozen disorders included in these screening programmes besides PKU and congenital hypothyroidism. In all cases, the main obstacles to successful screening were financial, logistical, and educational. Many programmes reported difficulties in obtaining dietary products and making contact for follow up of positive results. These problems are not unlike those faced in developed countries. In order for screening to be effective, it must function as a coordinated system of health care providers, testing laboratories, and fol-low-up. It is usually shaped by politics, geography and economics and must function within the confines of the political/social system that allows it to exist.

Velazquez found that screening was often performed in more than one location in developing countries, with little or no communications between programmes. These independent programmes were usually local rather than national, and often were located in private laboratories screening less than 10,000 infants annually. The sources of financial support varied and included private sources in at least one country, Brazil. There, it is funded by a society of parents of mentally retarded children[34]. Some countries have pursued creative financing through other means including a significant number of programmes receiving start-up assistance from the International Atomic Energy Agency (IAEA). This agency has also supported consult-ative review of its funded programmes by screening experts in order to improve and solidify these programmes. Extensive efforts supported by IAEA exist in a number of South and Central American countries, Mexico, and Thailand.

The programme in Thailand serves to exemplify the approach best suited for developing programmes[35,36]. Initially a plan was developed to establish laboratory testing procedures. A pilot programme was initiated to demonstrate a sufficient incidence of the disorder of interest, congenital hypo-thyroidism, to prove that the condition existed at a sufficient prevalence to support screening. Once the decision to screen was made, laboratory technology was transferred to the local testing areas and a field trial of the screening system initiated. All along the way, various education-al information was shared with appropriate persons, including physicians, politicians and consumers, and a final education effort took place at a national newborn screening conference prior to final programme im-plementation. The importance of a well planned programme and thorough education of all involved cannot be overemphasized. In Thailand, the initial pilot programme screened 21,504 newborns in 13 provinces. The overall incidence of congenital hypothyroidism was 1:1,792 with an increased incidence of 1:900 in iodine deficient areas of the country. Final implementation of a nationwide programme is now underway.

The goal of all newborn screening programmes are essentially the same. They include: (1) total participation of the eligible population; (2) notification and education of all parents (consumers); (3) prompt and reliable laboratory testing; (4) rapid follow-up of positive tests; (5) accurate diagnosis of confirmed positive cases; and, (6) appropriate treatment and counseling. Successful screening programmes also have similar characteristics including: (1) successful collaboration with other experienced programmes; (2) shared local resources; (3) education of health professionals and the public; and (4) political and economic support.

Future

The future of newborn screening is excitingly optimistic. More and more countries are developing screening programmes and those already developed continue to expand. Technical improvements impact both laboratory procedures and data handling. Computerization has progressed rapidly to the point that many programmes now receive electronic data from hospitals thus eliminating multiple data entry steps and improving data quality[37]. Laboratories have interfaced equipment result output directly into patient information databases so that automated, electronic downloading is available. Voice response systems allow health care workers to inquire about patient's laboratory results on a 24 hour basis and are often combined with faxing capability[38]. Patient follow-up can be documented in computer databases along with other patient data and the archived information linked to previous births to provide genetic histories[39].

In the screening laboratory there is emphasis on tandem mass spectroscopy[40] and DNA analysis[41]. In both cases, the current expense and limited utility to the principle screening disorders limits their utility to confirmatory testing. However, there is increased research effort directed at automated techniques and lowered costs for both. Currently DNA is used for confirmation of hemoglobin disorders, cystic fibrosis, medium chain acyl-coA dehydrogenase (MCAD) deficiency, and Duchenne muscular dystrophy. DNA testing has the advantage of not being influenced by the age of the patient (as in early discharge problems with other testing procedures) but has not yet been automated for analysis of disorders that might arise from any of a number of different mutations. It is likely that analysis strategies will be forthcoming to overcome these difficulties and that DNA analysis will be more widely favored for screening. Already this is causing legal, moral, and ethical concerns regarding the use of residual blood remaining on filter paper collection cards after newborn screening has been completed[20]. Newborn screening programmes must be careful to realize the important and complex arguments that are arising concerning this issue, and must develop policies to carefully protect the newborn screening services provided.

The definition of newborn screening is rapidly changing to one that views newborn screening as a system of identifying genetic and other health problems in newborns and other family members that leads to overall improvement in the public's health. programmes must be carefully oriented to improving the public's health in order to maintain the existence. Patients must be protected from possible abuses of a system that discovers genetic information for reasons not in the public's interest. Improved outcome in newborn morbidity and mortality must not be overlooked.

References

1. Garrod A. The incidence of alkaptonuria, a study in chemical individuality. Lancet 1902;2:1616.
2. Follig A. Uber aussheidung von phenylbenztraubensaure in den harn als stoffwech-selanomalie in verbindung mit imbezillitat. Hoppe Seyler Z Physiol Chem 1934;227:169–76.
3. Bickel H, Gerrard J, Hickmans EM. Influence of phenylalanine intake on phenylketonuria. Lancet 1953;2:812–13.
4. Bickel H, Gerrard J, Hickmans EM. The influence of phenylalanine intake on the chemistry and behavior of a phenylketonuria child. Acta Paediat 1954: 43;64–71.
5. Guthrie R, Susi A. A simple phenylalanine method for detecting phenylketonuria in large populations of newborn infants. Pediatrics 1963;32: 338–43.
6. Guthrie R. Screening for "inborn errors of metabolism" in the newborn infant — a multiple test program. Birth Defects Original Article Series IV 1962; 92–8.
7. Guthrie R. Routine screening for inborn errors in the newborn: "inhibition assays," "instant bacteria" and multiple tests. In Oster J, ed. Proc International

Copenhagen Congress on the Scientific Study of Mental Retardation. Copenhagen: Statens Andssvage Forsong, 1964:495–9.

8. Garrick MD, Dembure P, Guthrie R. Sickle-cell anemia and other hemoglobinopathies: procedures and strategy for screening spots of blood on filter paper as specimens. N Engl J Med 1973;288:1265–8.

9. Dussault JH, Laberge C. Thyroxine (T4) determination in dried blood by radioimmunoassay: a screening method for neonatal hypothyroidism. Union Med Can 1973;102:2062–4.

10. Dussault JH, Coulombe P, Laberge C. Preliminary report on a mass screening program for neonatal hypothyroidism. J Pediatr 1974;86:620–4.

11. Dussault JH, Parlow AF, Letarte J, et al. TSH measurements from blood spots on filter paper. A confirmatory screening test for neonatal hypothyroidism. J Pediatr 1976;89:550–2.

12. Pang S, Hotchkiss J, Drash AL, et al. Microfilter paper method for 17-hydroxy-progesterone radioimmunoassay: its application for rapid screening for congenital adrenal hyperplasia. J Clin Endocrin Metab 1977;45:1003–8.

13. Naruse H, Irie M (eds). Neonatal screening. Proceedings of the second international conference on neonatal thyroid screening, Tokyo, August 16–19, 1982 and the international symposium on neonatal screening for inborn errors of metabolism, Tokyo, August 19–21, 1982. Amsterdam: Excerpta Medica, 1983.

14. Therrell BL (ed). Advances in neonatal screening. Proceedings of the 6th International Neonatal Screening Symposium, Austin, Texas, 16–19 November 1986. Amsterdam: Excerpta Medica, 1987.

15. Wilcken B, Webster D (eds). Neonatal screening in the nineties. Proceedings of the 8th International Neonaal Screening Symposium. Leura, New South Wales, Australia: Kelvin Press, 1991.

16. Takasugi N, Naruse H (eds). New trends in neonatal screening. Proceedings of the 1st Asian Pacific regional meeting of the International Society for Neonatal Screening, Sapporo, Japan, 21–23 June 1993. Sapporo: Hokkaido Univ Press, 1994.

17. Farriaux J-P, Dhondt J-L. New horizons in neonatal screening. Proceedings of the 9th International Neonatal Screening Symposium and the 2nd meeting of the International Society for Neonatal Screening, Lille, France, 13–17 September 1993. Amsterdam: Excerpta Medica, 1994.

18. National newborn screening report. Infant Screening 1995;18–5.

19. Therrell BL, Panny SR, Davidson A, et al. U.S. newborn screening system guidelines: statement of the Council of Regional Networks for Genetic Services. Screening 1992;1:135–47.

20. Therrell BL, Hannon WH, Pass KA, et al. Guidelines for the retention, storage, and use of residual dried blood spot samples after newborn screening analysis:

statement of the Council of Regional Networks for Genetic Services. Biochem and Mol Med 1996; 57:116–24.

21. Meaney FJ, Kinney S, Kling S, et al. Assessing genetic risks — implications for health and social policy: response from the Newborn Screening Committee of the Council of Regional Networks for Genetic Services. Screening 1996;4:247–9.

22. Stern KS, Davis JG (eds). Newborn screening for sickle cell disease: issues and implications. Proceedings of the conference held in Washington, D.C., June 1993. New York: CORN Cornell University, Medical College, 1994.

23. Pass KA, Levy HL (eds). Early hospital discharge: impact on newborn screening. Proceedings of a conference held in Washington, D.C., March 31–April 1, 1995. Atlanta, Georgia: CORN, Emory University School of Medicine, 1996.

24. Freeman SB, Hinton CF, Elsas LJ (eds). Genetic services: developing guidelines for the public's health. Proceedings of a conference held in Washington, D.C., February 16–17, 1996. Atlanta, Georgia: CORN, Emory University School of Medicine, 1996.

25. Therrell BL, Aldis BG (eds). Proceedings of the 11th Natl Neonatal Screening Symp, Corpus Christi, Texas, September 12–16, 1995. Washington, D.C.: Assoc of State and Territorial Pub Hlth Lab Dir, 1996.

26. Therrell BL, Tuerck JM, McCabe ERB. Neonatal Screening systems in the United States — a critical review. In: Wilcken B, Webster D, ed. Neonatal screening in the nineties. Manly Vale, New South Wales, Australia: Kelvin Press, 1991: 18–24.

27. National Committee for Clinical Laboratory Standards. Blood collection on filter paper for neonatal screening programs — LA4-A2. Villanova, Pennsylvania: NCCLS, 1992.

28. American Academy of Pediatrics, Committee on Genetics. New issues in newborn screening for phenylketonuria and congenital hypothyroidism. Pediatrics 1982;69:104.

29. American Academy of Pediatrics, Committee on Genetics. Newborn screening for congenital hypothyroidism: recommended guidelines. Pediatrics 1987; 80:745.

30. American Academy of Pediatrics, Committee on Genetics. Newborn screening fact sheets. Pediatrics 1989;11:20–35.

31. American Academy of Pediatrics, Committee on Genetics. Newborn screening fact sheets. Pediatrics 1989;11:20–35.

32. American Academy of Pediatrics, Committee on Genetics. Issues in newborn screening. Pediatrics 1992;89:345–9.

33. Velazquez A. Neonatal screening in countries with socioeconomic developmental problems: results of an international inquiry. In: Farriaux J-P, Dhondt J-L, ed. New horizons in neonatal screening. Amsterdam: Excerpta Medica, 1994:301–7.

34. Schmidt BJ, Vargas PR, Martins AM, et al. PKU screening in Brazil. In: Farriaux J-P, Dhondt J-L, ed. New horizons in neonatal screening. Amsterdam: Excerpta Medica 1994:329–31.

35. Charoensiriwatana W, Janejai N, Tankananond W, et al. A pilot programme for neonatal screening in Thailand. In: Takasugi N, Naruse H, ed. New trends in neonatal screening. Sapporo: Hokkaido Press, 1994:23–5.

36. Charoensiriwatana W, Janejai N, Krasao P, et al. The establishment of national neonatal screening programme in Thailand. In: Therrell BL, Aldis BG, ed. 11th Natl Neonatal Screening Symp, Corpus Christ, Texas, September 12–16, 1995. Washington, D.C.: Assoc of State and Territorial Pub Hlth Lab Dir, 1996:1–4.

37. Porter LJ. A remote demographic data entry system (RDES) for newborn screening programs in Ohio. In: Skeels MR, Buist NRM, Tuerck JM, ed. Proc 6th Natl Neonatal Screening Symp, Portland OR, May 22–25, 1988. McLean, VA: ASTPHLD, 1988:48–50.

38. Pass KA, Schedlbauer LS. Automated telephone access to newborn screening information. In: Hofman L, ed. Proc 9th Natl Neonatal Screening Symp, Raleigh, NC April 7–11, 1992. McLean, VA: ASTPHLD, 1993:63–66.

39. Therrell BL. An optical disk archiving system applied to newborn screening. In: Hofman L, ed. Proc 9th Natl Neonatal Screening Symp, Raleigh, NC April 7–11, 1992. McLean, VA:ASTPHLD, 1993:67–9.

40. Chace DH, Millington DS. Neonatal screening for inborn errors of metabolism by automated dynamic liquid secondary ion tandem mass spectrometry. In: Farriqux J-P, Dhondt J-L, ed. New horizons in neonatal screening. Amsterdam: Excerpta Medica, 1994:373–6.

41. Zhang YH, Therrell BL, McCabe ERB. Automation of molecular genetic screening. In: Farriaux J-P, Dhondt J-L, ed. New horizons in neonatal screening. Amsterdam: Excerpta, 1994:377–8.

Screening Programmes in the Asian Pacific Area

Neonatal Screening in Mainland China: Current Status and Future Plans and Proposals

Daming Ying*, Ruiguan Chen, Yongnian Shen, Jun Ye, Xiaodong Huang

*Department of Neonatal Screening, Shanghai Institute for Pediatric Research, Shanghai Second Medical University, 1665 Kong Jiang Road, Shanghai 200092, China. *Corresponding author.*

Abstract *In China there are about 21 million newborns each year, among them about 1,800 new cases of PKU (1/11,186.) and 2,500 new cases of CH (1/5873). We started our work on neonatal screening in 1981. But after 14 years only 4 big cities in China have a complete organization for neonatal screening having government support, clinical pediatricians, laboratory support and a network for collection of blood samples. The recovery rate 90% and total number of babies screened 300,000/year. Some other cities may have neonatal screening programmes, but the recovery rate is very low, %. There is no screening programme in most parts of China. This year, a Law on the Mother and Child Health Care proclaimed: neonatal screening programmes must expand progressively in the whole country. There are difficulties: regional government's determination to support the programmes and the financial conditions of this region. We propose that in developed cities or regions, such as those in southern and eastern China, the government must enforce the Law and pay emphasis on neonatal screening programmes. The price of screening tests must be controlled and be flexible. Reagents for screening must be available at a low price. There should be available pediatricians, national quality control programmes and collaboration of different screening programmes such as screening for PKU, CH and iodine deficiency in endemic areas.*

Introduction

Phenylketonuria (PKU) and congenital hypothyroidism (CH) are important genetic diseases in China leading to significant health problems. China is a big country, with a population of over 1.2 billion and a birth rate of 17.7 per thousand in 1994. At this rate of population growth there are about 21 million babies born in one year. This poses a big challenge for nationwide neonatal screening for those genetic diseases of high frequency.

Current Status

Beginning in the early 1980s, first the Shanghai Institute for Pediatric Research and then the Department of Pediatrics of Beijing Medical University started preliminary neonatal screening for PKU and CH, which were considered as the two most important diseases requiring neonatal screening in China. In the past 15 years, the Shanghai Institute of Pediatric Research have screened a total of 585,000 newborns for PKU and 234,000 for CH in Shanghai.

From 1992 to 1993, the WHO and the Ministry of Public Health sponsored a cooperative project for neonatal screening in 7 major cities in China. The total number of newborn infants screened was 234,000. Among them 40 CH and 21 PKU were identified: the incidence of CH was 1/5,873 and the incidence of PKU 1/11,186. The expected number of new cases of CH and PKU would be 3,575 and 1,770 respectively every year.

In 1994, we carried out a survey by questionnaire. We found that the total number of newborns screened in 17 cities in China was approximately 0.2 million. This represented only 1% of the infants born in that year in the whole country. The remaining 98–99% have not been studied. However, in 4 cities, Beijing, Shanghai, Tianjin and Guangzhou, the neonatal screening programme was systematically implemented and screening rates of 80 to 90% were achieved.

The reagents used for screening are of prime importance. A reagent kit with good quality and at a reasonable price is needed. At present, we are using the Guthrie bacterial inhibition assay (BIA) for PKU screening and four different methods: RIA, IRMA, DELFIA and ELISA for CH screening. The ELISA method was more sensitive than RIA, as evident by the incidence rates of CH which was increased from 1/7 082 to 1/1 139 in the screening programmes carried out by our Institute.

There are two brands of locally made low phenylalanine diet available in China. These products have been proved to be useful in the prevention of brain damage in PKU patients.

Future Plan and Proposals

In the "Law on Maternal and Infant Health Care" published in 1995, Article 24 stipulates that the neonatal screening programme is to be developed gradually in the whole China. To implement and fulfill the objective of this article we propose that:

1. A time table for expanding the nationwide neonatal screening programme has to be defined;
2. A national committee on neonatal screening should be organized in order to coordinate exchange of experiences on neonatal screening among investigators and supervise the quality of work;
3. A multi-professional team to be organized in every city or screening center to conduct neonatal screening; an ideal task force should consist of pediatricians responsible for the diagnosis and treatment; a network of maternal hospitals and obstetric departments in general hospitals; a screening laboratory with good quality and a number of qualified social workers. This professional team should be responsible directly to the local government;
4. A less expensive reagent kit of CH for nationwide use has to be developed;
5. A locally made low phenylalanine diet has to be provided at reasonably low price. Alternatively an special insurance system should be set up to cover the expenses for PKU treatment be developed;
6. In the case of CH screening, the work of maternity hospitals and the Department on Endemic Diseases Control should be coordinated closely.

Nationwide Survey of Clinical Features of Wilson's Disease in Japan

T Aoki[1,2] *, M Suzuki[1], Y Fujioka[1], N Shimizu[1], H Fuji[1], H Nakazono[1], C Kawase[1], Y Yamaguchi[1], S Arashima[2], I Matsuda[2], M Arima[2]

[1] *2nd Department of Pediatrics, Ohashi Hospital, Toho University School of Medicine, Tokyo, Japan.* [2] *Japanese Committee for Wilson's Disease of Health and Welfare Government, Japan. * Corresponding author.*

Abstract *Our study of Japanese Wilson's disease was aimed at the analysis of clinical features, estimation of the exact prevalence rate and early detection by mass-screening. We sent questionnaires to 5,228 clinics and hospital departments all over Japan. From 1990 to 1994, a total of 673 cases of Japanese Wilson's disease were investigated. The prevalence rate was 1 in 30,000 to 34,000 live-births in Japan. Among the patients, 52.2% were of the hepatic type (including fulminant and hemolytic sub-types) of Wilson's disease and 14.3% were of the presymptomatic type. The youngest age of disease onset of Wilson's disease with fulminant hepatic failure and hemolysis was 5 years old. In spite of the administration of various methods of treatments, many patients still died of fulminant hepatitis or severe neurological defect. We should establish useful methodology for detection of Wilson's disease at the presymptomatic stage as early as possible in screening programmes.*

Introduction

In Wilson's disease, biliary excretion of copper and its incorporation in ceruloplasmin are both severely impaired. Symptoms of liver dysfunction may occur in children over 8 years old or in young puberty and adolescence. Acute onset is surprisingly frequent and hemolysis is often pronounced. Neurological damages are more frequently found after puberty.

Inheritance of Wilson's disease is autosomal recessive. The incidence is 1 in 30,000 to in 100,000 live-birth[1,2]. The gene is located at chromosome 13q1–14.3. The protein belongs to copper transporting P-type ATPase family, similar to that of Menkes disease, which is an X-linked disorder in copper transport[3,4,5].

This study on Wilson's disease in Japanese was aimed at analysis of the clinical features, estimation of the exact prevalence rate and early detection of this disease by mass-screening.

Methods

To study the clinical features of patients with Wilson's disease, we sent out questionnaires to 5,228 clinics, and hospital departments or divisions of pediatrics, child neurology, neurology, psychiatry, internal medicine and gastroenterology all over Japan. This questionnaire included information on the age of disease onset, sex, family history, clinical types of Wilson's disease, first symptoms, serum ceruloplasmin and copper concentrations, treatment-lag, methods of treatment and management of the patients.

Results

In the 5 years from January 1990 to December 1994, 673 cases were collected and investigated. Return rate of the questionnaires was 41.2%. The prevalence rate of Wilson's disease was found to be about 1 : 30,000 to 1 : 34,000 live-births in Japan. Sex ratio of males to females was about 55 to 45 and the peak age of disease onset was 12 years (Fig. 1). The hepatic type of Wilson's disease, including the fulminant and severe hemolytic type, was 52.2%, hepato-neurologic type 18%, neurologic type 13.5% and presymptomatic type 14.3% (Table 1). The youngest patient of presymptomatic type detected by family screening was 18 months old and the youngest case with only slightly elevated serum AST and ALT was 2 years old. He was a presymptomatic case detected by chance. The most common age of patients presented clinically of the hepatic type was 9 years

Table 1 Distribution of the age of disease-onset of each type of Wilson's disease

Type at onset	0–5	6–10	11–15	16–20	20–30	31	Total numbers of patients (%)	
Hepatic	12	131	165	18	5	5	336	(49.5)
fulminant	1	14	14	0	0	0	29	(4.3)
with hemolysis	0	16	16	3	0	0	35	(5.2)
Hepato-neurologic	1	21	43	18	30	8	121	(18.0)
Neurologic	0	9	41	18	15	8	91	(13.5)
Presymptomatic	35	49	11	1	0	0	96	(14.3)
unknown	0	8	10	6	3	2	29	(4.3)
	48	218	270	61	23		673	(100)

old, and of the neurologic type 13 years old. Twenty-nine cases of ful-minant hepatic failure were investigated, but 18 died within a few weeks. Only 8 cases are still alive. Partial liver transplantation had been performed in 3 patients, 2 were successful, but 1 died. In 97% of patients with Wilson's disease in Japan, serum ceruloplasmin concentrations were reduced to below 20mg/100ml (Table 2).

Table 2 Serum ceruloplasmin level of patients with Wilson's disease and their parents

Distributions of serum Cp level (mg/100 ml)	Number of patients with Wilson's disease	Parents of Wilson's disease patients		
		father	mother	father & mother
0–4.9	316 (59.5) } 463 (87.2)	1 (1.0)	2 (1.0)	3 (1.0)
5–9.9	147 (27.7)	5 (2.7)	7 (3.6)	12 (3.2)
10–14.9	42 (7.9) } 55 (10.4)	23 (12.6)	18 (9.2)	41 (10.9)
15–19.9	13 (2.4)	59 (32.4)	49 (25.1)	108 (28.6)
20–24.9	5 (1.0) } 13 (2.4)	41 (22.5)	61 (31.3)	102 (27.1)
25.0	8 (2.0)	53 (29.1)	58 (29.7)	111 (29.4)
Total	531 (100)	182 (100)	195 (100)	377 (100)

Discussion and Conclusions

We found that Wilson's disease in Japan has an incidence rate of 1 in 30,000 to 1 in 34,000 live-birth. This is similar to the worldwide prevalence of Wilson's disease which is about 1:23,000[1,2].

In spite of various methods of treatments, many patients in our survey still die of fulminant hepatic failure with severe hemolysis, severe hepatic damage and severe neurologic deterioration with irreversible brain dys-function.

Our results showed that we should establish methodology useful for mass-screening of Wilson's disease at the presymptomatic stage as early as possible. Early detection is extremely useful for treatment of Wilson's disease to improve morbidity and mortality.

References

1. Scheinberg HI, Sternlieb I. Wilson's disease. Vol. XX. In: Smith LH, ed. Major problem in internal medicine. Philadelphia: WB Saunders, 1984:1–171.
2. Danks DM. Disorder of copper transport. In: Scriver CR, Beaudet AL, Sly

WS, Valle D, ed. The metabolic basis of inherited disease, 6th ed. New York: McGraw-Hill Information Service Co., 1989:1411–31.

3.   Yamaguchi Y, Heiny ME, Gitlin JD. Isolation and characterization of a human liver cDNA as a candidate gene for Wilson's disease. Biochem Biophys Res Commun 1993;197:271–7.

4.   Bull PC, Thomas GR, Rommens JM, et. al. The Wilson disease gene is a putative copper transporting P-type ATPase similar to the Menkes gene. Nature Genet 1993;5:327–37.

5.   Tanzi RE, Petrukhin K, Chernov L, et. al. The Wilson disease gene is a copper transporting ATPase with homology to the Menkes disease gene. Nature Genet 1993;5:344–50.

A Trial Study for Neonatal Screening System of Wilson's Disease in Japan Using Dried Filter Papers

Norikazu Shimizu[1] *, Tomoko Nagayama[1], Hiroki Nakazono[1], Yoshimi Fujioka[1], Junko Miki[1], Shuichi Hiyamuta[2], Tsugutoshi Aoki[1]

[1] 2nd Department of Pediatrics, Toho University School of Medicine, Tokyo, Japan.   [2] Idemitsu Kosan Co Ltd, Chiba, Japan.   * Corresponding author.

Abstract   In Japan, the incidence of Wilson's disease is estimated to be between 1 in 30,000 and 1 in 35,000 live-births. This rate is higher than other inherited metabolic diseases that are already screened by neonatal screening programmes (e.g. PKU, MSUD). Therefore, we are trying to establish a mass-screening programme for this disease. The holoceruloplasmin levels in the dried blood on filter papers were detected by an ELISA method using antiholoceruloplsmin monoclonal antibodies. The trial study for neonatal mass-screening was carried out from 1993 to 1994 in 9 hospitals or institutions all over Japan. A total of 59,712 newborns were studied. The number of cases recalled for follow-up was 983 cases, the rate being 1.65%. There were 16 actual follow-up, a rate of 0.03%. Finally, 3 cases were identified to be hypoholoceruloplasminemia after three times reassessment. These 3 cases of hypoholoceruloplasminemia should be followed up for 2 to 3 years for confirmed diagnosis and treatment. We will continue this trial study for mass-screening of Wilson disease for several more years.

Introduction

Wilson's disease is an autosomal recessive disorder of copper metabolism, leading to accumulation of copper in several tissues, such as liver, brain, kidney, cornea and others. The three main features of the disease are liver dysfunction, extra pyramidal signs and Kayser-Fleischer ring. A worldwide frequency is between 1 in 35,000 and 1 in 100,000 live births, and this disorder is probably the most frequent cause of chronic liver disease in children[1]. However, Wilson's disease is treatable. The treatments with chelating agents, such as D-penicillamine and trienthylene tetramine, are established. The outcome with these treatments is mainly determined by the amount of damage which has occurred in the liver before treatment. A normal life span with normal health seems likely for patients diagnosed before cirrhosis or severe neurologic defects have developed. Early detection of this disease is extremely important. Therefore, a mass-screening programme is established by measurement of blood holoceruloplasmin levels in the neonatal period. In this report, we carried out the trial study of neonatal screening for Wilson's disease in Japan from 1993 to 1994.

Materials and Methods

A 10-question questionnaire was sent to 9 hospitals/institutions who work on Wilson's disease in Japan (Table 1). The survey addressed to the number of screened cases, positive cases, suspicious and diagnosed cases of Wilson disease. The base-line of serum holoceruloplasmin level was also included.

Table 1   The hospitals/institutions in Japan that were involved in the screening program

Groups	Name of institute	Area
1	Hokkaido Univ. and Sapporo City Sanitary Lab.	Hokkaido
2	Tohoku Univ.	Miyagi
3	Akita Univ.	Akita
4	Metropolitan Preventive Medical Society	Tokyo
5	Toho Univ.	Tokyo
6	Fukui Medical Coll.	Fukui
7	Univ. of Nagoya	Aichi
8	Tokushima Univ.	Tokushima
9	Kumamoto Univ.	Kumamoto

The holoceruloplasmin in dried blood on filter paper was detected by an immunoassay using anti-holoceruloplasmin monoclonal antibody[2]. Serum holocerulo-plasmin levels were measured by a sandwich ELISA method as described[3].

Results

Totally 59,712 newborns were screened. The number of positive cases in primary screening was 983. The frequency of positive cases in each hospital/institution ranged from 0 to 6.72%. The actual number of re-examined cases were 281 cases, account for 0.47% of the total. Among the re-examined cases 17 were found to be positive, which was 0.03% of the total. Sixteen of there 17 positive cases were further investigated, and finally 3 cases were identified to be hypoholoceruloplasminemia (Table 2).

Table 2 Results in each hospital/institution

	number of cases	positive	reinspection	positive in reinspection	re-reinspection
1	13537	9 (0.07%)	6 (0.04%)	0 (0%)	0 (0%)
2	7327	0 (0%)	6* (0.08%)	0 (0%)	0 (0%)
3	763	5 (0.65%)	5 (0.65%)	0 (0%)	0 (0%)
4	10984	738 (6.72%)	139 (1.27%)	9 (0.08%)	9 (0.08%)
5	818	4 (0.50%)	4 (0.50%)	0 (0%)	0 (0%)
6	5438	14 (0.25%)	0 (0%)	0 (0%)	0 (0%)
7	999	5 (0.50%)	5 (0.50%)	0 (0%)	0 (0%)
8	15846	97 (0.61%)	46 (0.29%)	8 (0.05%)	7 (0.044%)
9	4000	111 (2.00%)	70 (1.20%)	0 (0%)	0 (0%)
Total	59712	983 (1.65%)	281 (0.47%)	17 (0.03%)	16 (0.03%)

Each hospital or institution concluded her own base-line level of serum holoceruloplasmin for detection of hypoholoceruloplasminemia. The values ranged from 2.0 to 10.0 mg/100ml. Some hospitals used 2–5 percentile and mean-2SD.

Discussion

Because the serum total ceruloplasmin level is lower in the neonatal period than later in life, it is difficult to detect the newborn infants with Wilson's disease by ceruloplasmin measurement. However, serum holoceruloplasmin levels in newborn were significantly higher in Wilson's disease. We conclude that it is possible to detect Wilson's disease in newborn infant by immunoassay using antiholoceruloplasmin monoclonal antibody. This method is also useful for mass screening programmes. Our trial neonatal mass-screening programme detected 3 cases, which were 0.03% of the total of 59,712 newborn infants. The screening procedure was repeated 3 times. These cases should be followed up for 2 to 3 years to confirm diagnosis and effects of treatment. And we will continue this study for several more years.

References

1. Danks DM. Disorders of copper transport. In: Beaudet AL, Sly WS, Valle D, ed. The metabolic basis of inherited disease, 6th ed. New York: McGraw-Hill, 1989:1411–31.
2. Hiyamuta S, Shimizu K, Aoki T. Early diagnosis of Wilson's disease. Lancet 1993;342:56–7.
3. Fujioka Y, Aoki T, Shimizu N, et al. A new screening method for Wilson's disease by measuring blood caeruloplasmin level. In: Farriaux JP, Dhondt JL ed. New horizons in neonatal screening. Amsterdam: Excerpta Medica, 1994: 285–8.

Neonatal Screening for Glucose-6-phosphate Dehydrogenase Deficiency in Hong Kong

KK Lo[1], ML Chan[1], Ivan FM Lo[1], Stella SL Lai[1], Kitty CK Li[1], Patricia Hung[2], STS Lam[1] *

[1] *Neonatal Screening Unit, Clinical Genetic Service, Department of Health, Cheung Sha Wan Jockey Club Clinic, Shamshuipo, Hong Kong.* [2] *Neonatal Screening Laboratory, Institute of Pathology, Department of Health, Kwong Wah Hospital, Waterloo Road, Kowloon, Hong Kong.* * *Corresponding author.*

Abstract   *Hong Kong is geographically located at South East Asia, 97% of the population being ethnic Chinese. G6PD is a very common condition affecting the local people and population screening is justified. In 1984, the Central Genetic Neonatal Screening Unit was established as part of the Clinical Genetic Service in Hong Kong. The Unit screened for G6PD deficiency and congenital hypothyroidism in babies born at government hospitals and maternal and child health clinics. For screening purpose, blood was taken from the placental part of the umbilical cord immediately after delivery. This procedure ensured a high coverage and compliance. Affected children were counselled by appropriate medical personnel (community nurses, obstetric nurses, nurses at the Central Genetic Neonatal Screening Unit and nurses at maternal and child health centre) and a G6PD deficiency card together with education pamphlets were issued. All cases were traced by the Central Neonatal Screening Unit to ensure appropriate action was taken. From April 1984 to December 1994, a total of 432,153 babies (223,696 male and 208,457 female) were screened which represent 100% of the target population. G6PD deficiency was detected in 4.47% male and 0.27% female newborns.*

Introduction

Glucose-6-phospate dehydrogenase (G6PD) deficiency is a common condition affecting the southern Chinese population. Children with this condition are healthy with normal life expectancy. However, when provoked by certain drugs, chemicals or food, severe haemolysis may occur. When this occurs in the neonatal period, the resulting hyper-bilirubinemia may cause kernicterus with subsequent mortality and mental handicap.

Hong Kong is geographically located in South East Asia, with 97% of the local population being ethnic Chinese. G6PD deficiency is a very common condition. Previous studies in Hong Kong had showed that the condition affected 3% to 6% of the local males[1,2,3]. The medical implica-tion and the high incidence of G6PD deficiency would justify the implementation of a neonatal screening programme for early detection of this condition.

Methods

The neonatal screening programme for G6PD deficiency was imple-mented in Hong Kong in March 1984, together with neonatal screening programme for congenital hypothyroidism. The programme covered most of the babies delivered in the public institutions. By 1995, it covered 10 hospitals administered under the Hospital Authority of Hong Kong and 6 government maternity homes which represent the majority of all newborns born in the public sector.

For G6PD deficiency screening, 2.5 ml of cord blood was taken at birth at the placental side to an EDTA bottle and transported to the neonatal screening laboratory. G6PD deficiency was detected by the fluorescent spot test during the initially phase of the screening programme but later a quantitative assay was used for more reliable and objective results.

All cases of G6PD deficiency were reported to the Central Genetic Neonatal Screening Unit. Parents of affected children were contacted by telephone and by mail. Genetic counselling was given by appropriate medical personnel (community nurses, obstetric nurses, nurses at the Central Genetic Neonatal Screening Unit and nurses at maternal and child health centres). They were also given education phamplets and a G6PD deficiency card which included information on drugs, chemicals and food to be avoided. The Central Genetic Neonatal Screening Unit was respon-sible for tracing of patients to ensure all appropriate action to be taken.

Results

During the period from April 1984 to December 1994, a total of

432,153 live-births were screened for G6PD deficiency (223,696 males and 208,457 females) which represented 100% of the target population. G6PD deficiency was detected in 9,990 males and 578 females, which represented 4.47% and 0.27% of the population screened respectively.

Discussion

The incidence of G6PD deficiency for males in our study is 4.47% which is similar to that of previous studies. However, the incidence in females in this study is 0.27%, which is lower than that of another study performed in 1985[4]. The differences may be attributed to different sample size and different methodology for the G6PD assay.

During the past decade, we witnessed a marked decrease in mortality and morbidity caused by neonatal hyperbilirubinemia. Kernicterus, which used to be a major threat to neonates, is now almost unknown in the local population. The improvement in treatment of the condition by phototherapy and exchange transfusion is the major contributing factor. The role of the neonatal screening programme is to prevent neonatal haemolysis by avoiding provoking agents and to alert the neonatologist of the condition so that early intervention will be given to high risk babies. We conclude that neonatal screening programme for G6PD deficiency contributes towards prevention of mortality and mental handicap in the local population.

References

1. Chan TK, Todd D, Wong CC. Erythrocyte glucose-6-phosphate dehydrogenase deficiency in Chinese. Brit Med J 1964;2:102.
2. Lai HC, Lai MPY, Leung KSN. Glucose-6-Phosphate dehydrogenase deficiency in Chinese. J Clin Path 1968;21:44–7.
3. Yue PCK, Strickland M. Glucose-6-phosphate dehydrogenase deficiency and neonatal jaundice in Chinese male infants in Hong Kong. Lancet 1965;1:130–51.
4. Fok TF, Lau SP, Fung KP. Cord blood G-6-PD activity by quantitative enzyme assay and fluorescent spot test in Chinese neonates. Aust Paed J 1985; 21:23–5.

Implications of Antenatal HIV Screening

SS Lee

AIDS Unit, Department of Health, 5/F Yaumatei Jockey Club Clinic, 145 Battery Street, Kowloon, Hong Kong.

Abstract *Perinatal transmission is one of the routes through which HIV (human immunodeficiency virus) can be passed on from an infected mother to her newborn baby. Antenatal HIV screening offers one way of exposing the potential risk before a baby is born. Such screening, however, carries wide-reaching implication in view of its technical limitation and social impacts:*

(a) Antenatal HIV antibody testing has the intrinsic limitation of only identifying maternal infection instead of transmission. The average risk of perinatal infection is 15%–40%

(b) A positive HIV result carries with it social stigma and psychological stress. The need of maintaining confidentiality and providing counselling should be considered beforehand.

(c) Treatment is available to minimize the risk of perinatal transmission if maternal infection can be diagnosed. The best time to implement such treatment is still not known.

(d) Diagnosis of HIV infection in a newborn is often difficult because of the presence of circulating maternal antibody.

In view of the complexity of the issues involved, it is crucial that antenatal HIV testing is offered as a voluntary investigation. Counselling and social support should be available as an integral component of the testing system.

Introduction

There are three major routes of transmission for HIV, the human immunodeficiency virus — sexual contact, blood exposure, and from an infected mother to her child. Perinatal infection has become more important in recent years following a world-wide trend of heterosexual transmission. The risk of an infected mother passing on the virus to her new-born child ranges from 15% to 40%. Infection may occur before birth, during delivery or breast-feeding.

The HIV Test

Detection of HIV infection in the new-born is difficult because of the presence of circulating maternal antibody. In practice, HIV infection is diagnosed if the antibody test remains positive 18 months after birth, or when the infant has developed complications due to the underlying immunodeficiency. Other techniques like the HIV antigen test, polymerase chain reaction (PCR) or viral cultures may be useful in confirming a diagnosis. Their routine use for diagnosis remains to be established. On the other hand, antenatal HIV antibody testing has the intrinsic limitation of being able to identify only maternal infection but not transmission.

Preventing Perinatal HIV Transmission

The best means of preventing perinatal HIV transmission is to ensure that the mothers, or women of child-bearing age, are not infected in the first place. Preventive education and behavioural modification are therefore of primary importance.

Numerous studies have addressed the methods of minimizing the risk of HIV transmission from an infected mother to the baby. It is generally accepted that breast feeding should be avoided if safe artificial formula product is available. The effectiveness of caesarean section to prevent transmission remains a controversy. The use of antiretroviral treatment has drawn much attention following encouraging results released in 1994. According to the American study ACTG176[1], perinatal infection can be minimized by two-thirds if zidovudine is offered to the mother during the second and third trimester, followed by intravenous administration in the intrapartum period and oral feeding if the syrup preparation to the baby for six weeks after delivery.

The announcement of the ACTG results has changed the practice of health care workers in counselling HIV infected pregnant women. The United States Public Health Service[2] now recommends routine HIV counselling and voluntary testing for all pregnant women. In Hong Kong, the Scientific Committee on AIDS[3] has also revised its recommended guidelines on the management of paediatric HIV infection in line with similar principles. However, it must be noted that treatment is available only if maternal infection is diagnosed. The best timing and protocols for effective treatment are still not known.

Trends of HIV Epidemic and Perinatal Infection

World-wide, sexual transmission has accounted for three-quarters of all HIV infections known to date. With the rising trend of HIV transmission in the heterosexuals, perinatal infection would naturally become more prevalent. About 15,000 HIV infected babies were born in the United States between 1978 and 1993. An estimated 1,630 infants from 6,530 HIV infected women were born in the year 1993[4]. In Hong Kong, 59 of the 602 reported infections have occurred in women. Although the number is small, the rise in incidence is still alarming. The Department of Health has so far recorded 8 pregnancies involving HIV infected mothers. Two babies have been born with the virus. An estimated 136 HIV+ infants would have been born in Hong Kong by the year 2000[5].

With the adoption of new strategies, it is possible that the number of perinatally infected infants can be kept to a minimum. It is clear, however, that parallel development of public education, promulgation of professional guidelines, as well as training of health care staff are all crucial in minimizing the HIV problem in our society.

References

1. Conner EM, Sperling RS, Gelber R, et. al. Reduction of maternal-infant transmission of human immunodeficiency virus type 1 with zidovudine treatment. New Eng J Med 1994;331:1173–80.
2. Recommendations of the US Public Health Service Task Force on the use of zidovudine to reduce perinatal transmission of human immunodeficiency virus. MMWR Morb Mortal Weekly Report 1994;43(RR-1):1–20.
3. Guidelines of management of HIV infection in children. Hong Kong: Scientific Committee of the Advisory Council on AIDS, 1995.
4. Davis SF, Byers RH, Lindegren ML, et. al. Prevalence and incidence of vertically acquired HIV infection in the United States. JAMA 1995;247:952–5.
5. Chin J. Estimation and projection of HIV infection and AIDS cases in Hong Kong. AIDS Scenario & Surveillance Research Project Report, December 1994.

Management of
Screening Programmes

Management of Screening Programmes

Dianne Webster

National Testing Centre, P O Box 872, Auckland, New Zealand.

Abstract *Management of screening programmes can be discussed only when the scope and aims of the "screening programmes" is defined. In public health terms the aim of a screening programme is to reduce the morbidity and mortality from the condition screened for, so programmes consist of policy formation, funding, specimen collection and submission, laboratory, follow-up, treatment and audit aspects. The laboratory component may be considered as a clinical chemistry laboratory and the principles of laboratory management applied, however screening laboratories generally have a smaller number of less complex tests and a bigger number of samples than most clinical chemistry laboratories and this affects staff issues such as the appropriate mix of skills. There are increased demands for accuracy in screening programmes since tests are generally not done in duplicate and, since "well babies" are screened there is no clinical history to aid in result interpretation or detection of incorrect results prior to reporting. Other aspects of screening programmes are more complex to manage since these are often not under the control of, or co-ordinated by, a single person. Definition of the aims of the screening programme, audit of the extent to which the aims are achieved and feedback modification of all aspects of the programme to increase achievement are essential if screening programmes are to continue to expand in current financial climate.*

Management has implications of control, and control of having defined goals and a way of knowing whether the goals are being achieved. Performance indicators are a quantitative way of determining whether goals are met if they are carefully selected.

Management of screening programmes can therefore be discussed only when the scope and aims of the "screening programme" is defined. In public health terms the aim of a screening programme is to reduce the morbidity and mortality from the condition screened for. A number of aspects of the programme must be coordinated to achieve this aim, including policy formation, funding, specimen collection and submission, laboratory, follow-up, treatment and audit, yet few newborn screening programmes have all the above aspects under the control of one individual; in general screening policy is under the control of health funders; specimen collection within maternity services; treatment within paediatric services and the person often thought of as the manager of the screening programme is the manager of the screening laboratory. It is important that a single person or entity (possibly the screening laboratory manager or purchasing body) have an overview of all aspects of the programme, and develop political strategies to exert influence on the aspects which are not under direct control.

Policy development for newborn screening programmes can come from a variety of sources, which for the New Zealand programme includes the International Society for Newborn Screening and WHO guidelines (international); Council for Regional Genetic Networks (US); Human Genetics Society of Australasia and Australian College of Paediatrics Joint Newborn Screening Subcommittee; Ministry of Health Genetic Services and Newborn Screening Advisory Committee (local multidisciplinary committee); colleagues and informal networks.

Definition of the conditions screened for is necessary to count cases found and missed; the goalposts may be shifting as in the definition of PKU as hyperphenylalaninaemia needing treatment; the cutoff lines may not be clear as in screening for "saltwasting" CAH as distinct from "simple virilizing" CAH and the development of molecular techniques in cystic fibrosis screening and identification of affected infants from their mutation status has produced cases of CF without the "gold standard" of two positive sweat tests (although these can develop later). Individual screening programmes must develop clear definitions, and it is helpful for comparison of programme performance if these can be developed on a regional basis.

Staff management is especially difficult in screening laboratories. Management gurus give generally good advice about considering workers as motivated adults who should be treated fairly and with consideration but advice about rotation of tasks to give variety can only go so far in newborn screening laboratories with their small numbers of tests and large numbers of samples. This is easier in a situation where the screening laboratory is a section of a larger clinical chemistry laboratory. Because screening laboratories generally have only one sample from a well person, the clues available to pick up incorrect results prior to reporting in clinical chemistry laboratories are not available, so the screening laboratory staff must produce 100% correct results doing hundreds of TSH or phenylalanine measurements daily, most of them normal. This gives a considerable management challenge. In a relatively short time in screening laboratory management the techniques the author has found successful include delegating all decision making to the lowest possible level (including staff appointments, which are made communally); encouraging and rewarding desired behaviours; encouraging visits from PKU families; encouraging widespread use of the golden rule (do unto others ...) which is equivalent to consideration of all persons with whom one has interactions as customers.

Just as screening programme management is diverse, screening programme costs are difficult to accurately determine (as are the true costs of screening laboratories in many institutions). Screening laboratory costs under the general headings of staff, consumables and overheads are monitored within Auckland Healthcare and the performance indicators used include Tests done per full-time staff equivalent; staff costs as a proportion of total costs; costs compared to income (from selling tests to the health funder or clinical departments); number of stockturns annually. These provide useful comparisons within the screening laboratory from month to month but are less useful for comparisons between different laboratories within the organization.

Management of quality and performance standards in the screening programme again depends on defining what is required; the definition of quality as fitness for purpose is useful in this context. The screening laboratory can provide performance indicators to other parts of the screening programme such as number (%) of infants born who are screened; number (%) of samples not suitable for testing; number (%) of infants in whom appropriate follow-up was achieved; age at which diagnosis was made or age at which treatment was started as well as test sensitivity, specificity and positive predictive value. The latter performance indicators reflect performance within the screening laboratory as well as outside it. Within the laboratory, completion times for testing, time taken to reporting, number of tests needing to be repeated, performance in quality assurance programmes (especially using blinded samples) and other measures can be used of laboratory performance. Laboratory accreditation by an outside body can provide an indication of laboratory performance, however it is important to remember that most laboratory accreditation (for instance ISO9002) provides an audit of systems and process and that provision of a quality screening laboratory depends also on definition of appropriate screening policies and practices.

In 1994 our PKU screening had the following performance — 55 441 cards were received from 55 905 infants; 26/26 requested second samples were received. No cases of PKU or hyperphenylalaninemia were identified and none are known to have been missed. Testing of 99.5% of samples was completed in 4 calendar days or less and 5/6 blind QA samples at a level of 250 μmol/L (the cutoff level) were detected. The laboratory is Telarc — ISO9002 accredited.

In summary screening programme management is difficult as the different aspects of screening programmes are often not under the control of one person or organization. Screening laboratory management is similar in many ways to management of other laboratories but some consideration must be given to the particular characteristics of screening laboratories.

Management and Results of Mass Neonatal Screening in Lithuania

Vaidutis Kucinskas*, Vaclovas Jurgelevicius, Loreta Cimbalistienc, Dalia Jusciene, Marija Smirnova, Dalia Zamkauskiene

*Human Genetics Center, Vilnius University, Santariskiu 2, 2021 Vilnius, Lithuania. * Corresponding author.*

Abstract *Nationwide newborn screening for phenylketonuria (PKU) and congenital hypothyroidism (CH) was introduced in Lithuania in 1975 and 1993 respectively. The results are as follows: (1) 907,168 newborns were tested for blood phenylalanine levels; 85 PKU patients were detected; (2) 70,617 newborns were screened for CH; 16 cases of CH and 47 cases of transient hyperthyrotropinemia were diagnosed. Prevalence rates of PKU and CH in the Lithuanian population of newborns are 1:10,600 and 1:4,413 respectively. A system for the management of PKU and CH cases is in action in Lithuania at the Human Genetics Center (Vilnius). Genotype/phenotype correlation of PKU patients offers a possibility to predict the clinical outcome of PKU and to optimize dietary therapy.*

Introduction

Systems for managing phenylketonuria (PKU) and congenital hypothyroidism (CH) are introduced in Lithuania to prevent severe mental retardation and disability by early diagnosis and treatment. A diet low in phenylalanine (Phe) and replacement therapy by L-thyroxine are used for the treatment of PKU and CH respectively.

Methods

Mass neonatal screening for PKU   Different methods have been applied for estimation of blood Phe level, starting with Effron[2] and Guthrie[3]. In 1993, a fluorometric method was introduced for Phe estimation in filter paper blood disks[4]. Fluorescence was measured in a microplate fluorometer FLUOROSKAN II (Labsystems, Finland).

Mass neonatal screening for CH   TSH concentration was measured by enzyme immunoassay with fluorometric detection[5]. The cut-off value is 20 mIU/L blood (values up to 20 mIU/L were considered as normal). The CH diagnosis was based on the elevated TSH and decreased, T_4, T_3 or FT_4 concentrations in serum at the time of the first follow-up after the screening.

DNA analysis   PKU patients' DNA samples were screened for the presence of the following mutations in the PAH gene: R408W, R158Q, R261Q, IVS12nt1, IVS10nt546, Q232Q, and G272X.[6] DNA extraction, RFLP analysis and haplotype assignment were performed as described elsewhere.[7,8] Exons 5, 7 and 12 of PAH gene were amplified by the polymerase chain reaction.[9] ^{32}P-ASO probes were used for hybridization followed by stringent washing. Single-strand conformation polymorphism (SSCP) at the PAH locus were analyzed according to Labrune et al.[10]

Treatment and follow-up of the patients with PKU and CH   All newborns were tested for PKU and CH within a week after birth. In the case of blood Phe concentration >150 μM or blood TSH concentration >40 mIU/l, the parents and the child were invited to the Human Genetics Center (HGC) (Vilnius) for the verification of the diagnosis. The parents were counseled on dietary, medical and health insurance aspects. The aim of dietary treatment of PKU patients was to maintain plasma Phe level within the limits of 120–460 μM for preschool children and <700 μM for adults. Patients' IQ was measured by Wechsler Intelligence Scale for Children.[11] CH patients' treatment with L-thyroxine was started at 1–1.5 months of age. Recommended initial dose was 8–10 μg/kg body weight per day. Thereafter the dose was chosen individually on the basis of thyroid hormones and TSH serum levels analyzed by radioimmunoassay.

Results and Discussions

In our programme 907,168 newborns were screened for PKU between 1975 and 1995. At present we have 85 registered PKU patients and 4–5 newborns with PKU are identified every year. The incidence of PKU in the Lithuanian newborn population is estimated to be 1:10,600.

The mean patient's age at introduction of Phe-low diet was 21 ± 15 days. The satisfactory concentration of plasma Phe (>460 μM) was exceeded in 25% of the cases due to irregularities of dietary management. Subjects with the "worst" dietary control (average Phe concentration >800 μM) had mean IQ = 39 (mental retardation). In case of the "best" control (average Phe concentration <480 μM) intelligence quotient was higher. Other investigations were carried out to elucidate the relationship between phenylalanine hydroxylase (PAH) gene mutations, pretreatment Phe levels, mean of year Phe medians, and intellectual outcome. It was observed that pretreatment Phe level was higher in the case of PAH locus genotype R408W/R408W or R408W/R158Q (in comparison to other genotypes investigated). Our findings suggest that homozygosity for the mutation R408W leads to a severe clinical form of PKU.

The independent effects of four variables on IQ SD scores (age at start of treatment, diagnostic Phe concentrations, average Phe concentrations during treatment, genotype) were examined by multiple regression (Table 1). IQ SD scores showed no association with higher Phe concentrations at

Table 1 Multiple regression: IQ SD score and factors associated with pretreatment Phe concentration, average Phe concentration during treatment, and genotype (dependent variable: SD IQ).

Parameter	Estimate	T* for HO: Parameter = 0	Pr > T	Std Error of Estimate
AST[†]	−0.02983553	−4.40	0.0001	0.00678002
PPhe[‡]				
490–1200	−36.90407881	−4.73	0.0001	7.80772869
1200–2400	−42.00351873	−12.40	0.0001	3.38834573
2400<	−52.49387333	−5.64	0.0001	9.30362743
AST	−0.02285313	−3.60	0.0009	0.00635043
MPhe[§]				
301–400	−14.71440600	−0.90	0.3752	16.39810620
401–500	−18.20586531	−1.92	0.0621	9.46983353
501–600	−31.51726849	−4.71	0.0001	6.69700369
601–700	−44.99909487	−9.49	0.0001	4.74419003
701–800	−48.43309644	−8.68	0.0001	5.58190389
801–900	−48.13410697	−4.64	0.0001	10.37380584
901–1000	−36.48345658	−3.14	0.0033	11.63323414
1001<	−55.67709181	−10.19	0.0001	5.46592813
AST	−0.02621965	−3.66	0.0008	0.00715903
Genotype				
R408W/?	−43.93006732	−5.56	0.0001	7.89925589
R408W/R158Q	−37.44846236	−6.34	0.0001	5.90407049
R408W/R408W	−47.10111352	−11.56	0.0001	4.07413743

* T — Student's *t* statistics
[†] *AST* — age of start treatment
[‡] *PPhe* — pretreatment Phe concentration
[§] *MPhe* — mean of year Phe concentration medians

diagnosis. The influence of average Phe concentration and genotypes on IQ SD scores was statistically significant. genotype/phenotype correlation offers a possibility of predicting the clinical outcome of PKU and optimizing dietary therapy.

Nationwide neonatal screening for CH was introduced in Lithuania in 1993. Out of 70,617 newborns screened for CH from 1 August 1993 to 1 November 1995, 63 babies were found to be positives and required closer examination. Out of these, 16 cases of CH and 47 cases of transient hyperthyrotropinemia were detected. The incidence of CH in Lithuania 1:4,413 according to the results of our screening programme.

References

1. Lichter-Konecki U, Rupp A, Konecki DS, et al. Relation between phenylalanine hydroxylase genotypes and phenotypic parameters of diagnosis and treatment of hyperphenylalaninaemic disorders. J Inher Metab Dis 1994;17:362–5.
2. Guthrie R. Blood screening for phenylketonuria. J Am Med Assoc 1961;178:863.
3. Effron ML, Young D, Moser WH, MacCready RA. A simple chromatographic screening test for detection of disorders of amino-acid metabolism. N Engl J Med 1964;270:1378–83.
4. Gerasimova NS, Steklova IV, Tuuminen T. Fluorometric method for phenylalanine microplate assay adapted for phenylketonuria screening. Clin Chem 1989;36:211–5.
5. Tuuminen T, Rakkolainen A, Welin M-G, et al. A rapid fluorometric enzyme immunoassay for the determination of neonatal TSH from blood spots. Clin Chim Acta 1991;202:167–78.
6. Kuèinskas V, Jurgelevièius V, Cimbalistienë L, Holmgren G. Distributions of phenylalanine hydroxylase mutations and haplotypes in Lithuanian phenylketonuria patients. Hum Hered 1994;44:110–3.
7. Lidsky AS, Ledley FD, DiLella AG, et al. Extensive restriction site polymorphism at the human phenylalanine hydroxylase locus and application in prenatal diagnosis of phenylketonuria. Amer J Hum Genet 1985;37:619–34.
8. Güttler F, Ledley FD, Lidsky AS, et al. Correlation between polymorphic DNA haplotypes at phenylalanine hydroxylase locus and clinical phenotypes of phenylketonuria. J Pediatr 1987;110:68–71.
9. DiLella AG, Huang WM, Woo SLC. Screening for phenylketornuria mutations by DNA amplification with the polymerase chain reaction. Lancet 1988;1:497–9.
10. Labrune P, Melle D, Rey F, et al. Single-strand conformation polymorphism

for detection of mutations and base substitutions in phenylketonuria. Am J Hum Genet 1991;48:1115–20.

11. Wechsler D. Manual for the Wechsler Intelligence Scale for Children — Revised. New York: The Psychological Corporation, 1974.

Ethics of Neonatal Screening

Magnus Hjelm

Department of Chemical Pathology, The Chinese University of Hong Kong, Shatin, Hong Kong.

Abstract *Principles for the justification of neonatal screening of genetic disease are considered in this brief review. Similar considerations apply to prenatal and predictive screening of genetic disorders.*

Ethics can be defined as "system of principles of conduct". In the context of neonatal screening three parties could influence the formulation of such principles, (i) the neonate, (ii) the parents/family, and (iii) the society in the form of medical/legal professions and the community at large including the politicians.

The neonate should be the first subject to be involved in decisions about neonatal screening, but for obvious reasons the influence on decision making is in the order society, parents/family, neonate in most societies. The opinion by "society" is usually and initially represented by the medical profession, later to be translated into legislation, but views expressed by parental organizations are playing an increasingly important role in representing the position of the neonate, influencing politicians as makers of policy and law.

Shortly after the introduction of neonatal screening for phenylketonuria in the 1960s a "system of principles of conduct" was put forward by health professionals[1]. The system incorporated three criteria, (i) the urgency of early diagnosis where therapy was available, (ii) the technological feasibility of introducing neonatal mass screening, and (iii) the ratio for cost and benefit with regard to identify positive cases.

Based on these criteria four groups were identified, i.e. *Group 1*: neonatal screening recommended, all criteria fulfilled, therapy available (e.g. phenylketonuria), *Group 2*: neonatal screening not recommended despite therapy being available, because of lack of method for mass screening (e.g. aminoacidurias), *Group 3*: neonatal screening not recommended in high risk groups with fulfilled criteria because non-urgency of making the diagnosis (e.g.haemoglobinopathies), *Group 4*: neonatal screening not recommended because of doubtful benefit of early diagnosis and therapy (e.g. histidinaemia). Over the years quite a few disorders, initially not considered for neonatal screening, have been moved into the first group. Recent examples are screening of disorders, involving disturbances in the metabolism of amino acids, organic acids and fatty acids, which are treatable, and where analysis of blood spots at low-cost (per test) by mass spectrometry is now available[2]. Still the original classification has served well over a period of more than twenty years and tribute should be paid to those, who established the principles.

In view of recent developments a *5th Group* can be added to the scheme: Predictive neonatal screening for disorders presenting in childhood or adulthood (e.g. cystic fibrosis, Alzheimer's disease). This group can be said to differ from Group 2 and Group 4 because *genetic rather than biochemical investigations* are used for neonatal screening. This approach will allow homozygotes for a particular inherited disease as well as carriers to be identified, a difficult task using biochemical methods.

Opinions are emerging, addressing the ethics of carrying out predictive screening[3], based on a wide ranging debate. Examples of issues addressed are question such as "Do you agree that the following (parents, adoption agencies, medical practitioners) have the right to request that genetic testing (predictive or carrier status) be performed on a child — even if the result will have no direct health benefit for the child?". When this question was put to health professionals including geneticist, paediatricians, haematologists and co-workers substantial differences in attitudes were registered e.g. with 29% and 75% of co-workers and paediatricians, respectively, agreeing to parents making the decision.

Attitudes to detecting an inherited handicap vary with the type of handicap, e.g. about 20% in the general population felt that predictive screening was required for "low intelligence", whereas about 70 to 90% supported such screening for cystic fibrosis and Down's syndrome[4]. Presumably such figures to a degree reflect the general awareness of the nature such disorders in the population. Attitudes in families and among support groups vary substantially, as reflected in contradictory views such as "family uncertainty about the future is reduced" vs "predictive screening should not be done just for the parents' piece of mind", "parental expectation of the child's behaviour become altered" vs "testing will destroy the innocence of childhood" and "doctors should be able to refuse tests in order to protect the child" vs "doctors should have no say in the matter".

With such diverse opinions it is not surprising that the political machinery, claiming that "the Law is the society", is moving into the area of predictive screening, including prenatal and neonatal screening, with the aim to become the formal arbitrator of what is ethical in terms of accepted conduct. When that happens, substantial differences in medical practice will, no doubt, emerge between countries, as is the case in many other areas of medicine, the position of abortion being a prime example. Still financial constrains may directly and indirectly be the ultimate principle of conduct, directly because public funding for neonatal screening programmes will not be forthcoming, indirectly because the general public is either not sufficiently informed or misinformed about a very complex matter.

Collecting views from children and young adults with inherited disorders would be of special importance for formulating principles of conduct for neonatal screening. What do those children, who have been diagnosed with a hereditary disease, clinically expressed or not at birth, thing about neonatal screening, when they reach their reflecting age? Surprisingly little is known about the answers to this crucial question, which should be of equal importance to formulating principles of conduct with regard to both prenatal and neonatal diagnosis of inherited disorders.

References

1. Colombo JP, Hammersen G, Bickel H. Recommendations for newborn screening. In: Bickel H, Guthrie R, Hammersen G, ed. Neonatal screening for inborn errors of metabolism. Berlin, Heidelberg, New York: Sprinder-Verlag, 1980:315–6.
2. Chace DH, Hillman SL, Millington DS, Kahler SG, Roe CR, Naylor EW. Rapid diagnosis of maple syrup urine disease in blood spots from newborns by tandem mass spectrometry. Clin Chem 1995;41:62–8.
3. The genetic testing of children. Report of a working party (Clarke A, chairman) 1994. Clinical Genetics Society, Clinical Genetics Unit, Birmingham Maternity Hospital, Edgbaston, Birmingham B15 2TG, United Kingdom.
4. Focus: every child a perfect child. New Scientist 1995; 28 October: 14–17.

Studies on Inherited Metabolic Diseases

Maple Syrup Urine Disease (MSUD): Molecular Defect and Clinical Management

Ichiro Matsuda

Department of Pediatrics, Kumamoto University School of Medicine, Kumamoto 860, Japan.

Abstract   *Maple syrup urine disease (MSUD) is an autosomal recessive disease caused by a deficiency in any of the subunits (E1α, E1β, E2) of the branched chain α-ketoacid dehydroxylase complex (BCKDH). Since 1977, 36 Japanese patients with MSUD were identified by mass screening. Six died and the other 30 were followed while on specially prescribed diets. Among the 15 patients that we had studied, 8 had the classic type (leucine tolerance <600 mg/day) and 7 the non-classic type (intermittent, intermediate). BCKDH activity was 1.4 ± 1.7% in classic and 5.6 ± 3.0% in non-classic cases. Complementation study and gene analysis showed that 7 (3 classic, 4 non-classic) had E1α deficiency, 4 (all classic) E1β deficiency and 4 (2 classic, 2 non-classic) E2 deficiency. Only 2 identical mutant alleles were found in 2 families, one with E1α (A209T) and the other with E1β (11 bp dell) deficiency. All others were heterogeneous. Western analysis showed that missense mutations in the highly conserved codon of BCKDH and pyruvate dehydrogenase complex in other species, such as R115W, T209A in E1(gene, and frame shift mutations generating early and downstream stop codon generally result in classic MSUD with a severe reduction in the associated subunits (E1α + E1β or E2) of BCKDH. IQ or DQ was 69.0 ± 16.7 in the classic and 93.9 ± 10.7 in the non-classic MSUD patients.*

Introduction

Nationwide newborn mass-screening was started in 1977 in Japan. In this programme phenylketonuria (PKU), maple syrup urine disease (MSUD), homocystinuria, galactosemia were included. Congenital hypothyroidism and adrenal hyperplasia were added to the programme in

1979 and in 1989 respectively. From 1977 to 1993, approximately 22,000,000 babies were born in Japan, and during the last 5 years almost 100% of newborn babies have been tested by mass-screening, and approximately 90% of them have been followed up. The incidence of each metabolic disorder is listed in Table 1, indicating the incidence of PKU, MSUD, homocystinuria and galactoaemia in Japan to be from one-half to one-tenth of those in USA and in Germany respectively.

Clinical features of MSUD

Three different phenotypes have been distinguished in MSUD on the basis of clinical features: classic, non-classic (intermittent and intermediate) and thiamine dependent types. The patients with MSUD identified by mass-screening programmes were either of the classic or the non-classic type. No newborn infant has been diagnosed as the thyamine responsive type of MSUD so far in Japan. The IQ or DQ scores of the MSUD patients who were having dietary therapy ranged widely from 40 to 120 as shown in Fig 1. It is noted that the mean of IQ scores (82 ± 24) of these MSUD patients was apparently lower than that of the PKU patients who were also

Figure 1

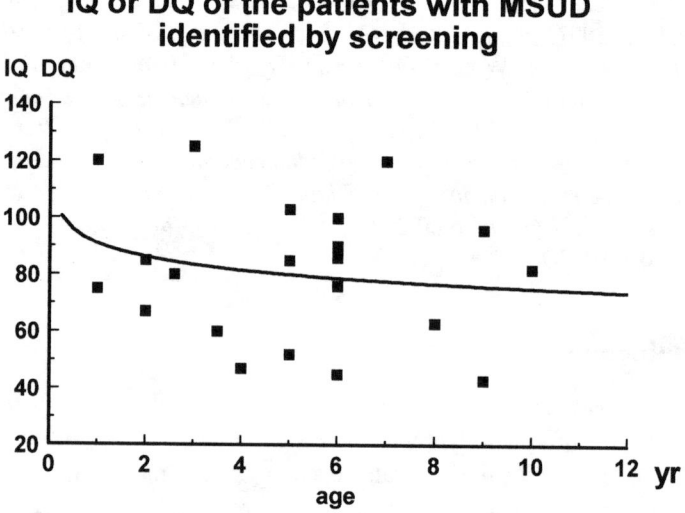

Table 1 Number of tested infants by newborn mass-screening of inborn errors of metabolism

	Live birth	Number of tested infants	Rate (%)
1977–1988	18,083,220	10,196,894	89.6
1989	1,241,717	1,255,187	101.1
1990	1,216,388	1,219,509	100.3
1991	1,220,933	1,230,449	100.8
1992	1,206,340	1,217,853	101.0
1993	1,194,475	1,206,219	101.0
Total	24,163,037	22,326,111	92.4

identified by screening programmes and were treated with dietary therapy (94 ± 15). Similar observations have been reported in Germany, the IQ or DQ scores being 74 ± 14 in MSUD and 101 ± 12 in PKU.

Biochemical and molecular aspect of BCKDH complex

The branched chain amino acids of valine, leucine and isoleucine enter the cells by specific transport system. They are either used for protein synthesis or converted to respective α-ketoacids by a cytosolic amino transferase. The branched chain keto acids enter the mitochondria, followed by decarboxylation through the activity of the branched chain keto acids dehydrogenase (BCKDH) enzyme complex. This complex is composed of three components; branched chain α-keto acid decarboxylase (E1), dehydrogenase (E2) and dihydrolipoyl dehydrogenase (E3). The E1 component is further composed of the E1a and E1b submits. MSUD is caused by the deficiency of either E1a, E1b or E2.

A full-length human E1a cDNA encodes for 445 amino acids and the E1a gene contains 9 exons and spans at least 55kb. A full-length E1b encodes 392 amino acids and the E1b gene contains 10 exons and is over 100kb length. A full-length of human E2 cDNA encodes 477 amino acids and the gene contains 11 exons and spans approximately 68kb.

Biochemical and molecular analysis of MSUD patients found at newborn screening

Since 1977, 36 patients with MSUD were identified by mass-screening in Japan. Six died and the other 30 survived and were followed up while on specially prescribed diet. Detailed follow-up study was carried out in 15 of them. Among these 15 patients 8 were the classic type (leucine tolerance <600 mg/day for maintaining plasma leucine level at 4.0 mg/dl) and 7 were the non-classic type (intermittent and intermediate). The relative BCKDH activity was 1.4 ± 1.7% in the classic group of patients and 5.6 ± 3.0% in the non-classic group when compared with normal subjects. Seven patients (3 classic, 4 non-classic) had E1a deficiency, 4 (all classic) E1b deficiency and 4 (2 classic, 2 non-classic) E2 deficiency as revealed by complementation study and gene analysis. Only 2 identical mutant alleles were found in 2 families, one with E1a (A209T) deficiency and the other E1b (11bp dell) deficiency. All other mutations were heterogeneous. Three of the 10 missense mutations were C-to-T transition in CpG dinucleotide (CpG to TpG or CpA). Missense mutations occurred in the highly conserved codons of BCKDH and pyruvate dehydrogenase complex in other species, such as R115W, A209T in E1a gene. Also detected were frame shift mutations due to a splicing abnormality, base insertion or base deletion, which generated stop condons early downstream. The latter usually resulted in classic MSUD. Western blot analysis of BCKDH revealed a severe reduction in the defective and associated submits (E1a + E1b or E2) of the enzyme complex in classic MSUD. IQ or DQ of these 15 patients were 69.0 ± 16.7 in classic and 93.9 ± 10.7 in non-classic types.

Comment

For nutritional control it seems to be much more difficult to maintain the plasma leucine concentration below 4.0 mg/dl in classic MSUD children than to keep the plasma phenylalaniane concentration below 6.0 mg ~ 8.0 mg/dl in PKU children.

Prenatal Diagnosis of Duchenne Muscular Dystrophy in China

Nianhu Sun

Beijing Union Medical College Hospital, Beijing, China.

Abstract   *Duchenne muscular dystrophy (DMD) is a disease of progressive muscle degeneration affecting the skeletal and cardiac muscles. The gene is located on the short arm of the X chromosome. Remarkable progress has been made in understanding of the dystrophin gene since its discovery in 1987. In the Peking Union Medical College hospital 71 DNA samples of unrelated affected children were analyzed by multiplex PCR using 14 sets of primers. 45 of them (63%) were found to have gene deletions. Two hot spots were discovered, exons 8–19 and exons 44–51. Short tandem repeat technique were used in 22 families to carry out RFLP analysis for carrier detection and prenatal diagnosis. A flow chart of prenatal diagnosis was designed. 55 cases of high risk pregnancies were studied. The dystrophin protein was studied by immunohistochemistry in 35 normal and affected fetuses. Fetal muscle biopsy under fetoscope were performed in 35 cases.*

Introduction

Duchenne muscular dystrophy (DMD), a disease of progressive muscular degeneration affecting the skeletal and cardiac muscles, begins early in life and usually ends in death by the second decade. It is a genetic disorder involving impairment in the production of dystrophin. The dystropin gene is located on the short arm of the X chromosome and the dystrophin protein is expressed and immunolocalized to the muscle membrane. It is a big gene spanning about 2.4 million base pairs. Direct DNA diagnosis and routine prenatal diagnosis are therefore difficult. The objective of this study is to use multiplex polymerase chain reaction (mPCR) and short tandem repeat (STR) techniques to carry out DNA diagnosis and prenatal diagnosis to identify dystrophin gene mutations. We also attempt to use histoimmunoassay to detect the dystrophin expression status of fetus and carrier.

Methods

Multiplex Polymerase Chain Reaction (mPCR) There were two groups of primers. One is nine pairs (for exons 4, 8, 12, 17, 19, 44, 45, 48 and 51) in one reaction system. The other is 5 pairs (for the promoter, exons 13, 43, 59, 52) in another reaction system. Totally 14 pairs of primers in two MTCR systems were used to detect dystrophin gene mutations in the DMD patients.

Short Tandem Repeat (STR) The STR technique was used to detect dystrophin gene mutations in the DMD families having no deletions. (Dr Chamberlain had reported 6 STR points having polymorphisms in the DMD gene). We have chosen four (CA)n points located in introns 44, 45, 49 and 50.

Immunohistopathology In our immunohistopathology investigation we used dystrophin antiserum P-20, Taq, which was a gift from Dr Bakker, to detect the fetal muscle of <12 weeks, 13–24 weeks and 25–40 weeks, in affected fetus diagnosed by DNA analysis.

Results and Discussion

In the 71 DMD/BMD cases, 63% (45/71) had gene deletions in one or more exons. In 55 cases of high risk pregnancies, 30 fetuses were STY positive. DNA analysis in 24 of the male fetuses showed that 9 of them were affected. The affected rate was 30%. Among the 25 females, 14 were studied by (CA)n Amp-FLP. Six were diagnosed as carriers. In the 6 female adults from DMD families requested for carrier study, 2 were identified as carriers by our DNA analysis.

The immunohistopathology analysis showed that in the 10 fetal muscle samples of <12 weeks, the stained dystrophin particles were in the cytoplasm. In 14 fetal muscle samples of 13–24 weeks, a proportion of the dystrophin moved to the sarcolemma. In 8 fetal muscle samples of 24–40 weeks, all dystrophin was located on the sarcolemma. In 6 women who had no family history but had delivered a DMD boy, their muscle samples showed the dystrophin network to be truncated. In 6 affected fetuses no dystrophin can be seen. These results suggested that DMD is active at birth despite the fact that clinical signs could not be recognized.

The mPCR protocol using 2 systems including 14 pairs of primers can detect 63% (45/71) of DMD cases with gene deletion. This is very close to the theoretical rate of gene deletion (65%). The deleted mutation has two hot spots in exons 8–19 and 44–51, which is consistent with Dr Caskey's findings.

Fetal muscle biopsy under the guide of fetoscopy is still an useful and reliable technique for prenatal diagnosis of DMD/BMD, particularly in situations when the DNA diagnostic technique is not available. The clinical history of the 71 affected DMO/BMD patients in this study was characterized by a steady deterioration of physical strength. The proximal muscle was usually affected first.

Conclusion

Sophisticated techniques such as mPCR and STR can now be used routinely used in clinics in China for DNA diagnosis and prenatal diagnosis. The discovery of two hot spots of deletion mutation has suggested the possible use of a new combination of 6 pairs of primers (for exons 19, 45, 48, 50, 51, 52). These oligonucleotide primers were synthesized and used in the Peking Union Medical College Hospital. The results obtained were clear, reproducible and therefore reliable. Our technical approach described here is simple and economical for use in developing countries.

Glucose-6-phosphate Dehydrogenase (G6PD) Deficiency: Mutation Detection and Its Implications

Veronica MS Lam

Department of Biochemistry, Faculty of Medicine, The University of Hong Kong, Hong Kong.

Abstract *Glucose-6-phosphate dehydrogenase (G6PD) deficiency is the most polymorphic human enzymopathy. About 3.4% of the world population is estimated to be at risk from its complications, the majority of these affected individuals live in the tropics and sub-tropics. Although most G6PD deficient individuals are asymptomatic, they are at risk for life-threatening haemolytic crises when triggered by certain external and environmental factors, such as drugs, some Chinese herbal medicines, or food, such as fava beans. It is also a globally and locally important cause of neonatal jaundice in newborns.*

Introduction

Glucose-6-phosphate dehydrogenase catalyses the first reaction in the pentose phosphate pathway and plays a major role in the regeneration of NADPH which is required for biosynthetic and detoxification purposes within cells, particularly in the metabolically restrictive red blood cells. Over three hundred variants have been characterized based on biochemical parameters in accordance with the WHO guidelines[1]. However, many ambiguities remain. Cloning of the G6PD gene followed by the use of different molecular detection methods led to the unraveling of about sixty different mutations, most of which are single nucleotide changes within the coding regions[2]. The results showed that heterogeneity at the DNA level is more extensive than previously envisaged[3,4] and that biochemical characterization has been misleading in some instances[3,4]. It is thus important to identify mutations at the gene level. The merits of the methods which had been used for detecting G6PD mutations will be reviewed. The implications of some of these mutations and their detection, in terms of relating the genotype to phenotype, will be discussed.

Single Strand Conformation polymorphism (SSCP)

Among the available detection methods, single stranded conformation polymorphism (SSCP) predominates as the method used to scan the gene for potential G6PD mutations. Sequencing the fragments which have been cloned into M13 or by directly sequencing the putative fragments led to the unraveling of many G6PD mutations[5,6]. SSCP has been widely used because it is sensitive and technically easy to handle. However, the fragments to be analyzed have to be short (~ 200bp) and it cannot attain 100% accuracy in detection of base changes. Some mutations could have been missed[7]. No theory at present can either predict the exact folded structure of single stranded DNA or accurately estimate the effect of structure on mobility in gel electrophoresis. One has to practically assess if the normal and mutation alleles of an amplified fragments would have different electrophoretic mobilities and therefore could be differentiated. Experience showed that the exon 2 mutation at nt 95 could not be identified[8] but when a different fragment was amplified (which encompasses this mutation) and electrophoresed, SSCP was able to differentiate the normal from the mutant allele.

Denaturing Gradient Gel Electrophoresis (DGGE)

Recently in our laboratory we have set up protocols in denaturing pelelectrophoresis (DGGE) as an alternative method to detect common G6PD mutations. At the same time we use these protocol to scan the gene for new mutations[9]. The electrophoretic patterns are distinctive for each of the mutant alleles studied and the heteroduplex provides a useful feature in identifying heterozygous females for an X-linked enzyme where enzyme assay may not be definitive. The computer algorithms MELT and SQHT programmes from Lerman can stimulate DNA melting profiles and predict the electrophoretic behaviour of partially melted DNA fragment, thus reducing the need to run empirical gels. With the amplification of a 40 bp GC clamp attached to one end of the fragment, detection can reach 100%. However, it requires a gradient gel.

Allele Specific Oligonucleotide Hybridization

So far only a few attempts, including our own, have been made to detect known mutations by allele specific oligonucleotide hybridization[10,11]. Our recent attempt with the use of digoxigenin labeled probes may enable the method to be adaptable for use in clinical service laboratories where large number of samples have to be analyzed. However, hybridization and washing conditions need to be established and carefully monitored. One other disadvantage is that this approach can only be used to identify defined mutations. Detection of novel mutations requires the use of other techniques.

Restriction Analysis

In many instances, a mutation often results in creating or destroying a restriction enzyme recognition site. Restriction digestion of the amplified fragment confirms a mutation which has been identified by other means. Very few of the Chinese G6PD mutations are amenable to such analysis. However, Chang et al. have successfully, by the use of a 3' mutagenesis primer, created an artificial restriction site for each of the common Chinese G6PD mutations[12]. This approach is simple and involves no hybridization. It has thus been adopted for use for diagnosis of these defined mutations in many laboratories[13].

Kinetic Studies

Results of attempts to correlate the identified molecular lesions with the kinetic and electrophoretic parameters of the GGPD variants, which differ in their degrees of deficiency and subsequently clinical severity (from class I to IV), have not been satisfactory[2]. In some cases, the electrophoretic and kinetic properties of the variants could be explained by the amino acid change(s) but in many others, the functionally important residues could only be inferred from kinetic data. Mutations which cause severe enzyme deficiency tend to cluster towards the 3' end of the gene and that a substantial proportion of these are found in exon 10[2]. Kinetic analyses of semi-purified enzymes from deleterious mutants led to the suggestion that the NADP+ (cofactor) binding site may be in this region[14] but recent structural studies fail to support this hypothesis[15]. It is clearly desirable to have recourse to the three dimensional (3-D) structure in order to understand the nature of the deleterious enzyme variants. However, this work has so far been hampered because sufficient amounts of purified sample of normal G6PD and variant G6PDs are difficult to come by. Recently we in our laboratory, as well as others, have succeeded in expressing normal and G6PD variant enzymes in *E. coli*. This paves the way towards determination of the tertiary structure of G6PD. Work has been initiated towards this goal. The ultimate aim is to be able to explain in detail the mechanism whereby a particular mutation in the G6PD gene causes a specific degree of G6PD deficiency.

Conclusion

Success in the detection of the responsible molecular lesions and identification of the G6PD heterozygotes would enable at-risk individuals to be unequivocally identified and counselled so that they would avoid the offending external agents. Advances in molecular detection methods could also be used to define more accurately the frequency of the mutations in G6PD deficient individuals in different ethnic populations. This will provide details of population genetics and epidemiology upon which health care policy and strategy are devised.

References:

1. Betka K, Beutler E, Brewer GJ, et al. WHO Scientific group: standardization of procedures for the study of G6PD, 1967. WHO Technical Report Series 366:1.
2. Vulliamy T, Beutler E, Luzzatto L. Variants of G6PD are due to missense mutations spread throughout the coding region of the gene. Hum Mutat 1993;2:159–67.
3. Vulliamy TJ, D'Urso M, Battistuzzi G, et al. Diverse point mutations in the human G6PD gene causing enzyme deficiency and mild or severe hemolytic anemia. Proc. Natl. Acad. Sci. 1988;85:5171–5.
4. Beutler E, Kuhl W, Vives-Corrores JL, Prchal JY. Molecular heterogeneity of G6PD A–. Blood 1989;74:2550–5.
5. Corcoran CM, Calabro V, Tamagnini G, et al. Molecular heterogeneity underlying the G6PD Mediterranean phenotype. Hum Genet 1992; 88:688–90.
6. Calabro V, Mason PJ, Filosa S, et al. Genetic heterogeneity at the glucose-6-phosphate dehydrogenase locus in southern Italy: a study on a population from the Cosenza district. Am J Hum Genet 1993;52:527–36.
7. Hayashi K. A method for detection of mutations. GATA 1992;9:73–9.

8. Lam VMS, Huang W, Lam STS, et al. Poster presentation entitled "Detection of the common Chinese mutations of G6PD deficiency by DGGE" at the Third "Mutation Detection" workshop, in Sweden, 1995, organized by HUGO.

9. Lam VMS, Haung W, Lam STS, et al. Rapid detection of common Chinese glucose-6-phosphate dehydrogenase (G6PD) mutations by DGGE. Genetic Analysis Biomolecular Engineering 1996;12:201–6.

10. Huang CS, Tang CJ, Huang MJ, Tang TK. Diagnosis of glucose-6-phosphate dehydrogenase (G6PD) mutations by DNA amplification and allele-specific oligonucleotide probes. Acta Haematol 1992;88:92–5.

11. Lam VMS, Huang W, Chow V, Johnson PH. Presented as a poster "A comparative analysis of three different methods used for identifying G6PD Chinese variations" at the 9th International Congress of Human Genetics in Brazil, 1996.

12. Chang JG, Chiou SS, Perng L, et al. Molecular Characterization of G6PD deficiency by natural and amplification created restriction sites: five mutations account for most G6PD deficiency cases in Taiwan. Blood 1994;80(4):1079–82.

13. Personal communication from Xie, J.S. Ph.D. thesis, Guangxi G6PD deficiency: mutations and clinical presentation, 1996.

14. Hirono A, Kuhl W, Gelbart T, et al. Identification of the binding domain for NADP$^+$ of human glucose-6-phosphate dehydrogenase by sequence analysis of mutants. Proc Natl Acad Sci 1989;86:10015–7.

15. Naylor CE, Rowland P, Basak AK, et al. Glucose-6-phosphate dehydrogenase mutations causing enzyme deficiency in a model of the tertiary structure of the human enzyme. Blood 1996;87:2974–82.

Phenylketonuria

A Study of 230 Cases of Phenylketonuria in China

Weimin Yu*, Xiaowen Li, Yaoyin Jin, Ming Sheng, Chun He, Li Xu, Fu Qia

*China-Japan Friendship Hospital, Beijing 100029, China. * Corresponding author.*

Abstract *We followed 230 cases of phenylketonuria (PKU) from October 1984 to December 1994. Treatment was provided for 20 cases (8.7% of total) identified by neonatal screening programme, when the children were less than 3 months old. 48 cases (20.9%) were treated when the children were 3–12 months of age. 162 PKU children (70.4%) were diagnosed when they were already more than 1 year old. Urinary pterins of 116 patients and erythrocyte dihydropteridine reductase (DHPR) activity of 86 patients were determined. Tetrahydrobiopterin loading test was carried out on 3 cases. One patient was found to be DHPR deficient and another diagnosed as 6-pyruvoyl-tetrahydropterin synthase deficiency. The phenylalanine hydroxylase (PAH) gene in 65 patients were analyzed by PCR-ASO and PCR-SSCP. Novel PKU mutations not reported in the Western populations were identified. To reduce the cost of treatment, locally-made PKU diet was produced in 1991 after repeated clinical trials. Now more than 150 PKU patients are taking locally-made low or free-phenylalanine (phe) diet which is supplemented with carnitine. The clinical results were satisfactory. Total and free carnitine blood levels in treated PKU subjects were significantly lower than those of controls (P < 0.01).*

Introduction

Phenylketonuria (PKU) is a common inherited disorder of amino acid metabolism. It is one of the major causes of hereditary mental retardation in children. A recent mass survey among newborn infants in China revealed that it occurs with an incidence of 1 in 16,500 live-births, similar to that in Caucasians but much higher than that in Japanese. In our hospital in Beijing, the neonatal screening programme was started in 1983. Two hundred and thirty cases of PKU from 21 provinces in China were under clinical and laboratorial observations from October 1984 to December 1994. In this report we describe their clinical, biochemical and molecular features.

Clinical observations

In 20 cases (8.7% of the total) of PKU identified by the neonatal screening programme, the treatment was given when the children were less than 3 months old, and they did not have the signs and symptoms of PKU. Among the rest of the 210 PKU children, 48 cases (20.9%) were detected and treated at the age of 3–12 months and 162 (70.4%) were diagnosed when they were more than 1 year old. All these 210 PKU children had some signs and symptoms of PKU. Mental retardation was found in 98% of them and various patterns of seizures in 24%. All of the 230 patients had hyper-phenylalaninemia, which was the basis of diagnosis.

Screening for tetrahydrobiopterin deficiency and differential diagnosis

Urinary pterins obtained from 116 PKU patients were measured by high performance liquid chromatography[1]. Dihydropteridine reductase (DHPR) activity in blood was determined in 86 cases and tetrahydrobiopterin (BH_4) loading tests were done in three of them. Among the 116 patients, two had hypotonia and convulsion and developed a progressive neurologic disorder despite adequate treatment for PKU. High concentration of neopterin but only traces of biopterin were found in the urine specimens of these two patients. Loading tests with BH_4 were carried out, and a rapid normalization of the elevated plasma phenylalanine level occurred within 4 hours after administration of 10 mg/kg body weight of BH_4. DHPR activity was nor-mal. Based on the above results, 6-pyruvoyl tetrahydropterin synthase (PTPS) deficiency was diagnosed for these two patients. Treatment and gene mutation analysis of the two cases are in process.

Molecular biology of phenylalanine hydroxylase

Defects in the Phenylalanine hydroxylase (PAH) gene in 65 classical PKU patients and their parents were analyzed by using polymerase chain reaction (PCR)-allele specific oligonucleotide (ASO) and PCR-single strand conformation polymorphism (SSCP). Novel PKU mutations which had not been found in the Western population were detected and identified by DNA sequencing.

Used of locally produced low phenylalanine diet

To reduce the expenses of treatment of PKU patients, a locally made PKU diet (bentongkang) was used in 1991 after repeated trials[2]. Three sister formulae were produced. Formula I is a complete diet for infants in which the phenylalanine (phe) level is 40 mg/100 gm powder; formula II and III are phe free for older children (formula II is complete diet; formula III is protein only). More than 150 cases of PKU have been taking locally-made phe diet. The clinical results were satisfactory. After conclusive use of the formula I or II for 2 to 4 days, the phe level in blood dropped to be within the reference range. Follow up for patients treated with bentongkong revealed that their physical development was normal and mental development was satisfactory.

Serum carnitine level in PKU patients under dietary treatment

L-carnitine is found in all mammalian tissues and is especially necessary for cells capable of utilizing fatty acids. Carnitine is required for the transport of fatty acids and reduced cellular carnitine may adversely affect the fatty acid oxidation. The PKU diet is a practically carnitine free diet because the protein-based supplementary formulae were carnitine free and the small amount of natural protein was of vegetable origin. Meat, egg and cow's milk, which are rich in carnitine are almost completely excluded. In order to evaluate the effects of the PKU diet on the distribution of carnitine, serum carnitine was determined in 15 PKU patients on diet (7 males and 8 females). They were aged 1 ~ 6 years with no clinical signs of carnitine deficiency, malnutrition or evidence of liver and renal dysfunction. Concentrations of total, free and esterified carnitine in blood, were found to be low in PKU patients under dietary treatment (Table 1). We propose that the PKU patients who are normal in their blood phenylalanine levels should be supplemented with carnitine.

Table 1   Serum carnitine level (μ mol/L; mean ± SD):

Carnitine	PKU (n = 15)	Control (n = 14)	P
Total	24.55 ± 5.32	45.95 ± 7.37	<0.01
Free	18.07 ± 5.58	30.84 ± 5.39	<0.01
Esterified	6.92 ± 3.42	15.11 ± 5.55	<0.01

Follow-up for PKU patients and study on early home intervention of PKU children

A total of 102 cases of PKU were treated with low-phenylalanine diet and were followed up by health workers[3]. The duration of treatment was 0.8–7.2 years. On the latest visit, their age ranged from 1 to 8 years and their physical development was normal. The level of blood phenylalanine was not significantly different among the 3 treatment groups, group 1 treated early at age 3 months, group 2 at 12 months and groups 3 older than 12 months. The DQ/IQ in group 1 (early treatment) was normal and higher than that in groups 2 an3 (treated more lately). The abnormality rate of electroencephalogram (EEG) in group 1 was the lowest (Table 2). These results again suggest that early diagnosis and early treatment for PKU patients are very necessary. China is a large country, and newborn screening has not been carried out in many regions. Most PKU patients coming to our hospital already have various degrees of mental retardation. To improve their mental development, early home intervention was given to 8 PKU patients with mild mental retardation for 6 months to 2 years. Their developmental quotient (DQ) and mental age in year were significantly improved (DQ elevated by 15 ~ 21). Their behaviour functions in motor

Table 2   DQ/IQ and EEG in different groups:

Group	Ages of starting treatment	n	DQ/IQ (mean SD)	EEG abnormal rate
1	~3M	19	94.5 ± 10.3* (82.6–109.4)	5.0 (1/19)*
2	~12M	37	69.3 ± 17.6* (32.7–97)	29.7 (11/37)*
3	>12M	46	41.8 ± 16.5 (25.4–82)	67.4 (31/46)

* Significantly different from another group P < 0.01

and language were also better than before. We suggest that early family intervention should be given to the PKU patients even though they are treated late. Their clinical conditions and development would certainly be improved. This measure is also effective and economical in our country.

Conclusions

1. Neonatal screening programme for PKU should be established in the whole of China as soon as possible.
2. Differential diagnosis should be made for classical PKU and BH4 deficiency in hyperphenylalaninemic individuals as early as possible.
3. To relieve the financial burden, we could use less expensive low-phenylalanine diet which was produced in China.
4. The phenylalanine-free formulae for PKU patients should be supplemented with carnitine.
5. Early home intervention for the late treated PKU patients is effective and beneficial for the development of the patients.

Acknowledgments

This project was supported by funds received from the Commission of Education of the People's Republic of China. We are grateful to Drs Hsiao KJ, Matsuda I and Huang SZ for their collaboration in laboratory work. We are also grateful to Dr Kitagawa T, Japan Snow Brand Milk products Co., Ltd., Japan Kyowa Hakko Kogyo Co., Ltd. and Japan Morinaga Milk Industry Co., Ltd. for their support and encouragement in our research on PKU.

References

1. Yu WM, Zhang JQ, Chang M, et al. A simple and sensitive method of determining urinary pterins for the differential diagnosis of hyper-phenylalaninemia. Chin J Med Genet 1992;9:294.
2. Yu WM, Xu L, Sheng M, et al. Clinical results of PKU treated with local-made formula. Proccedings of Third China Human Genetics Symposum, Dalian, 1994:329.
3. Sheng M, Yu WM, Xu L, et al. Inquisition about developmental quotient and early intervention of phenylketonuria children. Journal of China-Japan Friendship Hospital 1994;8:151.

Prenatal Diagnosis in 16 Pregnancies with High Risk of Phenylketonuria

Lifang Yuan[1]*, Shangzhi Huang[1], Huiyuen Lo[1], Binliang Fang[1], Tao Yang[1], Tao Wang[1], Nianhu Sun[2]

[1] *Department of Medical Genetics, Institute of Basic Medical Sciences, Chinese Academy of Medical Sciences,* [2] *Beijing Union Medical College Hospital, Beijing 100005, China. * Corresponding author.*

Abstract *Classical phenylketonuria (PKU) is the most common inherited metabolic disease resulting in severe mental retardation in childhood. It is caused by a deficiency of hepatic phenylalanine hydroxylase (PAH). Even though PKU can be treated effectively with low phenylalanine diet, some shortcomings do exist. Many parents seek for prenatal diagnosis. Since the PAH activity does not express in chorionic villi or amniotic cells, DNA analysis is the exclusive method for prenatal diagnosis of PKU. In northern China most PKU are caused by the point mutations occurred in exons 3, 6, 7, 10, 11 and 12 of the PAH gene. We use PCR-ASO hybridization, PCR-SSCP to detect the mutations and PCR-STR for linkage analysis in PKU families. 16 cases of prenatal diagnosis were performed. 7 fetuses predicted as normal were confirmed after birth. 5 predicted as affected were aborted by induction. One fetus predicted as affected was born PKU because the result of DNA analysis came too late. One pregnancy ended in spontaneous abortion. The outcomes of the rest of the pregnancies are still pending.*

Introduction

Phenylketonuria (PKU) is a common inborn error of metabolism with autosomal recessive inheritance. The prevalence in China is 1 per 12,000 live birth. Classical PKU is caused by deficiency of hepatic phenylalanine hydroxylase (PAH). Most untreated patients are severely mentally retarded[1].

There is no doubt that administration of a low-phenylalanine diet in early infancy prevents mental retardation. Unfortunately, most of these treated children are not entirely mentally normal, even though they have been under the strictest dietary control. The average I.Q. of these children are usually 12 to 17 points below that of their parents. They often manifest learning disabilities in school and behaviour abnormalities. Perhaps the most distressing problem involved with PKU is that of the potential for fetal damage and leading to mental retardation in offsprings of women with PKU. This syndrome, which includes mental retardation, microcephaly and possible cardiac anomalies. This phenomenun has been termed "maternal PKU". Low phenylalanine diet cannot totally prevent PKU. Many parents are seeking prenatal diagnosis. Prenatal diagnosis of PKU cannot be done by measuring phenylalanine level in the fetus, nor by measuring the PAH enzyme activity because these measurements would require a fetal liver biopsy. DNA analysis is already feasible for prenatal diagnosis of PKU[2,3] and has been shown to be reliable.

During the past five years, we have successfully accomplished prenatal diagnosis in 16 pregnancies with high risk of PKU. We used DNA technique and here we report the outware at our analysis.

Materials and Methods

Materials   5–10 ml blood was collected from members of 30 PKU core families. WBC were isolated by hypotonic ammonium chloride. For prenatal diagnosis, chorionic villi biopsy was performed at 8–12 weeks of pregnancy. Amniotic cells were collected at 16 weeks of pregnancy. DNA was extracted from the isolated WBC.

Methods   PCR (polymerase chain reaction), mediated ASO (allele specific oligonucleotide) blot hybridization, PCR-SSCP (single strand conformation polymorphism) were used to detect mutation in PKU families. PCR-STR (short tandem repeat) was used for linkage analysis.

PCR-ASO   The annealing temperature for PCR amplification of genomic DNA for PAH exon 7, 12, 6, 11,10, 3 was 53°C. PCR products were denatured, dotted onto Zetaprobe membrane. Hybridization with ^{32}P labelled normal and mutant ASO probe. Prehybridization and hybridization were carried out at 50–54°C and stringently washed at 50–57°C. The membrane was heated to dry and then exposed to X film.

PCR-SSCP   PCR amplification was the same as for PCR-ASO. PCR products were denatured at 96C for 5 minutes, and then applied to 8%

polyacrylamide gel containing 5% glycerol, electrophoresis at 600 V, 4 C–21C for 5–7 hrs. The gel was then subject to silver staining.

PCR-STR   STR lies 700 bp 3′ to PAH exon 3. It contains tandemly repeated (TCTA)n motifs, spans from 228–260 bp. There are 9 alleles at this site. The procedure was according to a previous report[4]. Prenatal diagnosis were of 10 cases were carried out by PCR-ASO alone, 3 cases by PCR-SSCP, 1 case by SSCP combined with ASO, and 1 case by using a combination of ASO and STR.

Results

16 cases of prenatal diagnosis with high risk of PKU was performed. 7 fetuses predicted as normal were confirmed after birth. 5 predicted as affected were ended in induced abortion of which 2 were confirmed by examination of placenta. One fetus predicted as affected was diagnosed to have PKU by the Guthrie test, blood Phe 20 mg%. One fetus predicted as normal ended in spontaneous abortion, the outcomes of the two predicted as normal are pending.

Discussion

The human PAH gene was isolated in 1983 by SLC Woo. It spans about 90 kb with 13 exons, codes for a protein of 451 amino acids. Most PKU are caused by point mutations in the PAH gene. Mutants R243Q, R413P, Y204C, Y356X, W326X and T111X are most common among PKU in Northern China and account for 62% of PKU mutations. Combined with PCR-ASO, PCR-SSCP, and PCR-STR techniques, we are able to make prenatal diagnosis in 80% PKU families. When using chorionic villi, samples shoud be cautiously processed to prevent contamination by maternal cells resulting in mistake of prenatal diagnosis.

Acknowledgments

This study was supported by the Chinese Ministry of Public Health and the Chinese Medical Board, USA.

References

1. Scriver CR, Clow CL. Avoiding phenylketonuria: why parents seek prenatal diagnosis. J Pediatr 1988;113:495.
2. Woo SLC, Lidsky AS, Guttler F, et al. Cloned human phenylalanine hydroxylase gene allows prenatal diagnosis and carrier detection of classical phenylketonuria. Nature 1983;306:151.
3. Fang BL, Yuan LF, Wang M, et al. Detection of point mutation of the phenylalanine hydroxylase gene and prenatal diagnosis of phenylketonuria. Chin Med Sci J 1992;7:205.
4. Goltsov AA, Eisensmith RC, Naughtan ER, et al. A single polymorphic STR system in the human phenylalanine hydroxylase gene permit rapid prenatal diagnosis and carrier screening for phenylketonuria. Hum Mol Genet 1993; 2:577.
5. Hayashi K. PCR-SSCP: A simple and sensitive method for detection of mutations in genomic DNA. PCR Method and Application 1991;1:34.
6. Brandt B, Greger V, Yandell D, et al. A simple and non-radioactive method for detecting the Rb1.20 DNA polymorphism in the retinoblastoma gene. Am Hum Genet 1992;51:145.

Detection of the Mutation Gene in Phenylketonuria and Prenatal Diagnosis by PCR-SSCP Combined with Silver Staining

T Yang[1] *, LF Yuan[1], SZ Huang[1], BL Fang[1], M Wang[1], NH Sun[2], SM Zhao[2], WHY Lo[1]

[1] *Department of Medical Genetics, Institute of Basic Medical Sciences, Chinese Academy of Medical Sciences, Beijing, China.* [2] *Beijing Union Hospital, Beijing, China.* * Corresponding author.

Abstract *We applied the single strand conformation polymorphism (SSCP) technique combined with silver staining to screen for mutations in the four exons of the phenylalanine hydroxylase (PAH) gene. After PCR amplification, the DNA fragments were separated by electrophoresis on polyacrylamide gel containing glycerol and visualized by silver staining. Three known missense mutations were detected, R243Q in exon 7 [CGA(Arg^{243}) $\rightarrow$ CAA(Gln)], Y356X in exon 11 [TAC(Tyr^{356}) $\rightarrow$ TAA(Ter)] and R413P in exon 12 [CGC (Arg^{413}) $\rightarrow$ CCC(Pro)]. These three are hot-spot mutations in Chinese PKU patients. Three abnormal DNA bands in exon 10 were detected by SSCP and were under further investigation. We have identified the PAH gene mutations in 11 PKU families. Prenatal gene diagnoses were successfully performed in 7 pregnancies at risk with PKU.*

Introduction

Classical phenylketonuria (PKU) is a common autosomal recessive genetic disorder, whose frequency is about 1 in 10000 among Chinese. PKU is primarily a consequence of a deficiency in phenylalanine hydroxylase (PAH) activity and untreated PKU patients develop severe mental retardation.

To establish easy, rapid and reliable methods to detect mutations in the PAH gene, we applied single strand conformation polymorphism (SSCP) combined with silver staining technique to screen for mutations in the four exons of the gene. The DNA regions examined were amplified by polymerase chain reaction (PCR).

Methods

Patients Fifteen Chinese PKU families were recruited for mutation analysis. Genomic DNA was isolated from peripheral blood samples of both parents and the affected children. Seven pregnancies at risk with PKU were chosen for prenatal gene diagnosis. Fetal genomic DNA was prepared from amniotic fluid cell or chorion villus. All the blood, cells and biopsy samples were supplied by the Beijing Union Hospital.

PCR amplification Primers for in vitro amplification of regions in exon 7, 10, 11 and 12 of the PAH gene were synthesized as described. PCR was carried out in a 50 µl reaction volume containing 0.5 µg genomic DNA, 100 µM of each dNTP, 125 ng of each primer, 2 units of Tag DNA polymerase (SABC), $1 \times$ Tag. buffer (50 mMKCl, 1 mMTris-HCl pH 9.0, 0.1% Triton X100). The PCR programme 30s of denaturation at 94°C, 30s of annealing at 53°C, 60s of extension at 72°C.

SSCP analysis 6 µl PCR product was diluted in 4 volume of loading buffer (95% formamide, 10 mMEDTA pH 8.0, 0.1% bromophenol blue, 0.1% xylene cyanol) and applied to 8% polyacrylamide gel containing 5% glycerol after 5 min of denaturation at 96°C. Electrophoresis was performed at 600 V at constant temperature which was different for each exon.

Silver Staining The gel was incubated for 10 min in solution I (10% ethanol, 0.5% acetic acid), 3–5 min in 0.2% AgNO3, and 5–10 min in solution II (1.5% NaOH, 1.08% formaldehyde).

Table 1   Results of mutation detection in 15 PKU patients

mutant	detected gene	mutant gene
E7aR243Q	30	12
E7b	30	1
E11 Y356X	30	4
e12 R413P	30	2
E10*	30	4
Total	30	23

* three kinds of abnormal band in E10 were shown as E10a, E10b and E10c

Figure 1 Detection of point mutations: R243Q(exon 7)(A), Y356X (exon 11)(B) and R413P (exon 12)(C) in PAH gene by SSCP technique. Prenatal diagnoses of family 1 at risk with PKU are shown in (A) and (B).

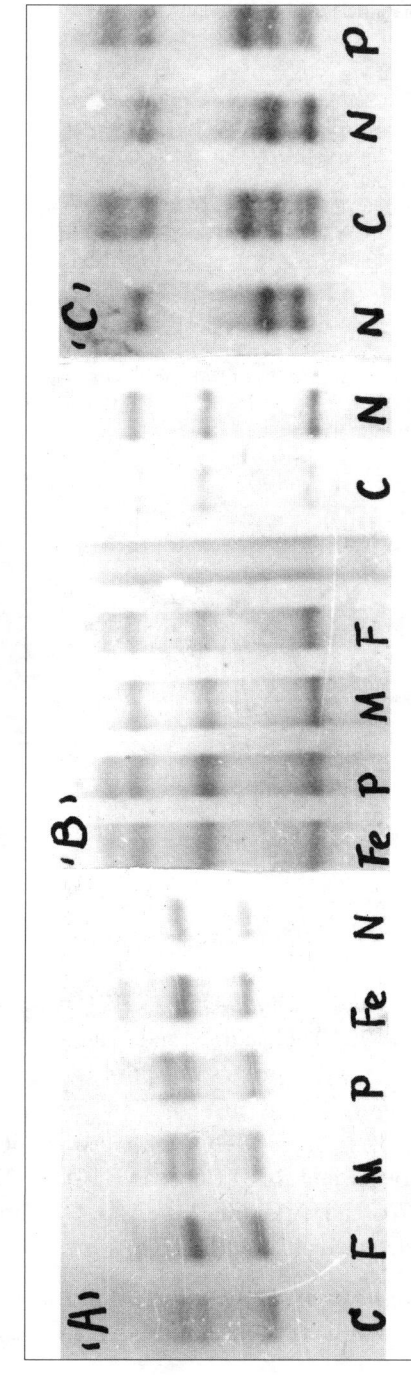

Table 2 Prenatal diagnosis of phenylketonuria

family no.	patient	fetus	confirmation
1	R243Q/Y356X	Y356X/Normal	normal, birth
2	Y204C/R243Q	R243Q/Y204C	affected, aborted
3	R243Q/R243Q	r243q/r243q	affected, aborted
4	R43Q?	?/Normal	normal, birth
5	Y204C/E10c	Y204C/Normal	normal, birth
6	R413P/Y356X	Y356X/Normal	normal, birth
7	R243Q/E7b	Normal/Normal	normal

Figure 2 SSCP analysis in exon 10 of PAH gene and results of prenatal diagnoses in
family 2 at risk with PKU. The symbols: E10a, E10b and E10c represent three
kinds of abnormal fragments in exon 10.

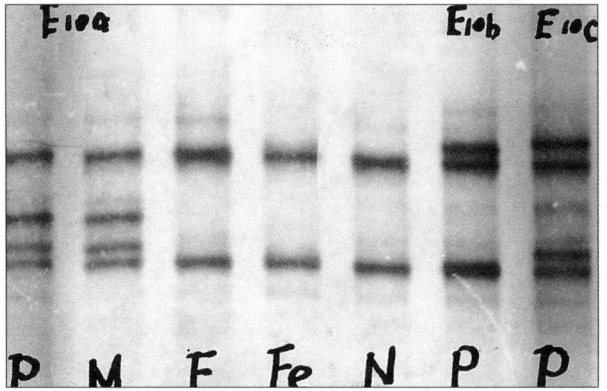

Results

Detection for PAH gene mutations in 15 PKU patients   We screened for
mutations in exons 7, 10, 11 and 12 and found seven abnormal patterns.
Known mutations were used as positive controls. Two varied
electrophoretic conformations in exon 7 were detected at 21C, one of
which is R243Q[CGA(Arg243) $\rightarrow$ CAA(Gln)]. Y356X[TAC(Tyr356) $\rightarrow$
TAA(Ter)] in exon 11 and R413[CGC(Arg413) $\rightarrow$ CCC(Pro)) in exon 12
were detected at 7°C and 28°C (Fig. 1 — A, B, C). Three abnormal patterns
in exon 10 were detected at 21°C (Fig. 2).

Prenatal gene diagnosis of PKU families   Prenatal diagnosis were carried
out in seven PKU families (Table 2, Fig 1-A, B, Fig 2)

Figure 3 Screening result of point mutation R243Q (exon 7) in a family at risk with PKU. Patient is homozygous for the R243Q mutation. His father and mother are heterozygous for the mutation.

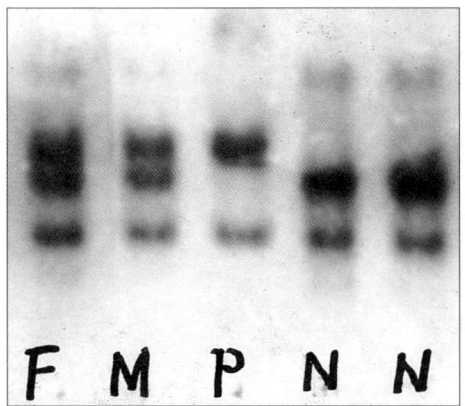

Abbreviations: C-dominate control; F-father; M-mother; P-patient; Fe-fetus at risk; N-normal individual

Discussion

We have applied the SSCP technique to screen for mutations in 6 exons of the PAH gene in PKU individuals. Although several experimental conditions were tested, the mutations in exon 3 and exon 6 did not give rise to conformation changes on electrophoresis. This is the disadvantage of SSCP technique.

However, nonradioactive PCR-SSCP has many advantages: (1) It is convenient and fast, and the possibility to have a false-positive is low. (2) It is economical and safe with silver staining instead of radioactive isotope.

The mutations we have detected by SSCP are hot spots of mutations in Chinese PKU patients. We have also made some technical improvement so that our procedure can be applied for mutation analysis and prenatal diagnosis of PKU. Our laboratory protocols are also capable of analyzing large numbers of samples.

The Fragile X Syndrome

Instability of the Trinucleotide Repeat in the FMR-1 Gene

Priscilla MK Poon, Calvin CP Pang*

*Department of Chemical Pathology, The Chinese University of Hong Kong, Shatin, Hong Kong. * Corresponding author.*

Abstract *The fragile X syndrome is the most common hereditary cause of mental retardation in Caucasian populations. Its occurrence has been reported in many other ethnic groups across the world including Africans, Indians, Japanese and Chinese. It is inherited in an X-linked semi-dominant modee with reduced penetrance and is caused by unstable expansion of a CGG repeat in the 5′ untranslated region of exon 1 of the FMR-1 gene. Such expansion has been shown to lead to hypermethylation of the promoter, abolishment of the FMR-1 gene expression and impairment in mental development of the affected individual. The CGG repeat sequence is interspersed with the AGG triplet, which is assumed to provide stability, the so-called anchorage effect, to the repeat sequence. The length of an uninterrupted CGG repeat sequence is related to unstable transmissions. Instability of microsatellites in the fragile X chromosome, notably the highly polymorphic FRAXAC2, may be associated with the CGG expansion. Haplotype studies involving the FRAXAC1 and DXS548 microsatellite markers, which have linkage disequilibrium with FMR-1, revealed exceedingly dominant fragile X associated alleles*

Diagnosis of the Fragile X Syndrome

The fragile X syndrome of mental retardation is one of the most common genetic diseases and the most common form of familial mental retardation. The chromosomal abnormality of an unusual constriction in the distal X chromosomes in affected males and carrier females was first described by Lubs in 1969[1]. The syndrome is characterized by mild to severe mental retardation, IQ from 70 to 30, facial dysmorphism, behavioural disturbances and macroorchism in 70% to 90% of the adult males[2]. The phenotypic features are subtle and variable, and therefore clinical diagnosis is unreliable. The conventional method of detection is the cytogenetic feature of an inducible folate-sensitive fragile site on the long arm of the X chromosome at Xq27.3[3]. Characterization of the fragile X locus and the FMR-1 gene in 1991 leads to establishment of DNA diagnostic methods[4]. Detection of the fragile X mutations by Southern hybridization and polymerase chain reaction provide direct diagnosis[5,6]. DNA analysis detects both affected individuals and carrier females and can be used for prenatal diagnosis.

The Mode of Inheritance

In 1983 a study of polymorphic DNA markers in the segregation of the X-chromosome in fragile X families have shown that phenotypically normal males can transmit the fragile X syndrome, the normal transmitting males[7]. Results of a large study on 206 families segregating for the syndrome have revealed the imbalance of the penetrance of the phenotype[8]. Daughters of normal transmitting males are almost at 100% risk of inheriting the fragile X mutation but are phenotypically normal, whilst daughters of normal carrier females have 50% risk of inheriting the mutation but 16% risk for mental retardation. The penetrance of mental impairment and risk of inheriting the mutation depends on the mental status of the mother if she is a carrier and upon the position in the pedigree. This unconventional pattern of X-linked inheritance is known as the "Sherman Paradox"[9].

The FMR-1 Gene

The mutation locus of the fragile X syndrome was localized at the fragile site FRAXA in Xq27.31[10,11]. The associated gene is the FMR-1 gene which consists of 17 exons spanning 38 kb with significant alternative splicing towards the 3′ end[12]. The fragile X mutation is the expansion of a CGG repeat located in the CpG island and at the 5′ untranslated region of the first exon of the FMR-1 gene. In affected fragile X individuals, there is abnormal DNA methylation in the CpG island which is associated with absence of FMR-1 expression[13,14]. The CGG repeat is polymorphic in normal human, ranging in size from 6 to 54 repeats with the most frequent allele of 29[15] or 30 repeats[6]. Alleles with approximately 45–55 copies are said to be in the "gray zone"[16]. Some of them are stably inherited while others are unstable and are expanded from generation to generation. The FMR-1 mutation can be a premutation or a full-mutation. Asymptomatic carriers, including normal transmitting males, their daughters and other unaffected carrier females, have the premutation with 50–230 copies of CGG repeats, with little or no somatic heterogeneity and with no abnormal methylation of the CpG island[10]. Premutations are not known to be associated with abnormal phenotype such as mental retardation[10,17]. All affected fragile X individuals have full mutation of more than 230 copies and abnormal methylation of the FMR-1 CpG island. Full mutations are associated with mental retardation in more than 90% of the affected males and 55% affected females. Full mutation individuals usually exhibit somatic variation of repeat length and up to 15% of them have premutations in some of their cells[5]. They are known as "mosaics"[10] and full mutation males have a significantly higher prevalence of mosaics than females, 12% against 6%[17].

Fragile X Gene Instability

Other factors have been shown to contribute to the unstable nature of the fragile X mutation. Within the CGG repeat sequence of the FMR-1 gene there are interspersed AGG trinucleotides which apparently provides anchorage of the repeat sequence and prevent slippage during replication process[18,19]. The interspersed AGG positions are highly polymorphic. In a study on 54 premutation individuals with 56–180 CGG repeats, 63% had no AGG and 37% had one AGG[20], while in 133 normal control subjects, 1.5% had no AGG, 25% had one, 71% had two and 3% had three. It is probable that normal individuals having their CGG repeats uninterrupted by AGG at the 3′ end or have 30–40 pure CGG repeats would have increased risks for expansion. Loss of AGG apparently destabilizes the CGG region.

There is strong linkage disequilibrium between FMR-1 alleles and nearby proximal microsatellite polymorphic markers including the FRAXAC1, FRAXAC2 and DXS548[21,22]. In one study on normal Chinese X chromosomes 90% of the 29 CGG repeat alleles had the FRAXAC1 152 bp allele against 41% of the 30 CGG repeat alleles[23]. In the Swedish population two haplotypes of the FRAXAC2 and DXS548 microsatellites accounted for 64% of fragile X chromosomes but only 14% of the normal chromosomes[24]. In the Japanese population a significant correlation existed between the CGG repeat number and the FRAXAC1 and 2 alleles[25]. Such striking linkage disequilibrium supports founder effect of the fragile X chromosomes in different populations[26].

The unique nature and complexity of the fragile mutation at the FMR-1 gene account for the peculiar pattern of inheritance of the syndrome. So far all known fragile X individuals and families carry the same gene mutation[15,27].

References

1. Lubs HA. A marker X chromosome. Am J Hum Genet 1969;21:231–44.
2. Hagerman RJ. Physical and behavioral phenotype. In: Hagerman RJ, Silverman AC, ed. Fragile X syndrome: diagnosis, research and treatment. Baltimore, USA: The Johns Hopkins University Press, 1991:3–68.
3. Sutherland GR. Fragile sites on human chromosomes: demonstration of their dependence on the type of tissue culture medium. Science 1977;197:265–6.
4. Verkerk AJMH, Pieretti M, Sutcliffe JS, et. al. Identification of a gene (FMR-1) containing a CGG repeat coincident with a breakpoint cluster region exhibiting length variation in fragile X syndrome. Cell 1991;65:905–14.
5. Rousseau F, Heitz D, Biancalana V, et al. Direct diagnosis by DNA analysis of the fragile X syndrome of mental retardation. New Eng J Med 1991;325: 1673–81.
6. Brown WT, Houck GE, Jeziorowska A, et al. Rapid fragile X carrier screening and prenatal diagnosis using a nonradioactive PCR test. JAMA 1993;270: 1569–75.
7. Camerino G, Mattei MG, Mattei JF, et al. Close linkage of the fragile X linked mental retardation to haemophilia B and transmission through a normal male. Nature 1983;306:701–7.
8. Sherman SL, Jacobs PA, Morton NE, et.al. Further segregation analysis of the fragile X syndrome with special reference to transmitting. Hum Gen 1985;69: 289–99.
9. Sherman SL. Epidemiology in fragile X syndrome. In: Hagerman RJ, Silverman AC, ed. Fragile X syndrome: diagnosis, research and treatment. Baltimore, USA: the Johns Hopkins University Press, 1991;69–97.
10. Oberle I, Rousseau F, Heitz D, et al. Instability of a 550-base pair DNA segment and abnormal methylation in fragile X syndrome. Science 1991;252: 1097–102.
11. Yu S, Pritchard M, Kremer E, et al. Fragile X genotype charcterized by an unstable region of DNA. Science 1991;252:1179–81.
12. Eichler EE, Richards S, Gibbs RA, Nelson DL. Fine structure of the human FMR-1 gene. Hum Mol Genet 1993;2:1147–53.
13. Hertz D, Rousseau F, Devys D, et al. Isolation of sequences that span the fragile X and identification of a fragile-X-related CpG island. Science 1991;251:1236–9.
14. Pieretti M, Zhang F, Fu YH, Warren ST, Oostra BA,Caskey CT, Nelson DL.

Absence of expression of teh FMR-1 gene in Fragile X syndrome. Cell 1991;66:817–22.

15. Fu YH, Kuhl DPA, Pizzuti A, et al. Variation of the CGG repeat at the fragile X site results in genetic instability: resoulation of the Sherman Paradox. Cell 1991;67:1047–58.

16. Park V, Howard-Peebles P, Skherman S, et al. Policy statement: American College of Medical Genetics. Fragile X syndrome: diagnostic and carrier testing. Am J Med Genet 1994;53:380–1.

17. Rousseau F, Hertz D, Tarleton J, et al. A multicenter study on genotype-phenotype correlations in the fragile X syndrome, using direct diagnosis with probe StB12.3: the first 2,253 cases. Am J Hum Genet 1994;55:225–37.

18. Eichler EE, Holden JJA, Popovich BW, et al. Length of uninterrupted CGG repeats determines instability in the FMR1 gene. Nat Genet 1994;8:88–94.

19. Snow K, Tester DJ, Kruckeberg KE, et al. Sequence analysis of the fragile X trinucleotide repeat: implications for the origin of the fragile X mutation. Hum Mol Genet 1994;3:1543–51.

20. Zhong N, Yang W, Dobkin C, Brown WT. Fragile X gene instability: anchoring AGGs and linked microsatellites. Am J Hum Genet 1995;57:351–61.

21. Richards RI, Holman K, Friend K, et al. Fragile X syndrome; genetic localization by linkage mapping of two microsatellite repeats FRAXAC1 and FRAXAC2 which immediately flank the fragile site. J Med Genet 1992;28: 818–23.

22. Zhong N, Dobkin C, Brown WT. A complex mutable polymorphism located within the fragile X gene. Nat Genet 1993;5:248–53.

23. Zhong N, Liu X, Gou S, et al. Distribution of FMR-1 and associated microsatellite alleles in a normal Chinese population. Am J Med Genet 1994; 51:417–22.

24. Malmgren H, Gustavson KH, Oudet C, et al. Strong founder effect for the fragile X syndrome in Sweden. Eur J Hum Genet 1994;2:103–9.

25. Richards RL, Kondo I, Holman K, et al. Haplotype analysis at the FRAXA locus in the Janpanese population. Am J Med Genet 1994;51:412–6.

26. Zhong N, Ye L, Dobkin C, Brown WT. Fragile X founder chromosome effects: linkage disequilibrium or microsatellite heterogeneity? Am J Med Genet 1994;51:405–11.

27. Rousseau F, Rouillard P, Morel ML, et al. Prevalence of carriers of premutation-size alleles of the FMR1 gene — and implications for the population genetics of the fragile X syndrome. Am J Hum Genet 1995;57:1006–18.

Normal FMR-1 Alleles in the Chinese Population

Priscilla MK Poon[1], Zhen Zhao[1], Chang H Yin[2], Xiang-qian Wu[2], Yu-xing Ni[2], Calvin CP Pang[1]*

[1] *Department of Chemical Pathology, The Chinese University of Hong Kong, Shatin, Hong Kong.* [2] *Faculty of Medical Laboratory Sciences, Rui Jin Hospital, Shanghai Second Medical University, Shanghai, China.* *Corresponding author.*

Abstract *The Fragile X syndrome is related to the number of trinucleotide CGG repeats at the 5' untranslated region of the causative FMR-1 gene. We have studied 994 normal X chromosomes from unrelated Chinese subjects in Hong Kong, Shanghai, Changsha and Dalian which are located in different parts of China. CGG repeats was analyzed by polymerase chain reaction and detected by hybridization with a ^{32}P labelled $(CCG)_5$ probe. A different distribution pattern of CGG allele size from the Caucasians is observed, it is a bimodal pattern and the most common CGG repeat allele is 29 against 30 in the Caucasians. Five alleles of more than 50 CGG repeats were detected, four of them in heterozygous females. There was no difference in the repeat pattern in subjects from the four Chinese cities, suggesting no geographical differences. Our data provides a foundation for screening of affected individuals and carriers of the fragile X syndrome in the Chinese population.*

Introduction

The fragile X syndrome is the most frequent familial form of mental retardation and is the commonest cause of mental retardation after Down's syndrome[1]. In Caucasian populations its prevalence is estimated to be 1 in 1250 males and 1 in 2500 females[2]. In affected adult males, the syndrome is characterized by mental retardation, macroorchidism, and behavioural anomalies such as autism[1,3]. Clinical features of female carriers are much less prominent, and only about 30% suffers from mild mental retardation[3]. The syndrome is associated with a folate-sensitive fragile site on the X-chromosome at band Xq 27.3[1]. Cytogenetic analysis of the X-chromosomes provides a standard method of detection but the test is positive only in a proportion of male or female carriers who are phenotypically normal[4,5]. An hypermethylated DNA region characterized by a high density of cytidine phosphate guanosine (CpG) dinucleotides has been revealed in the Fragile X site in Xq27.3 of Fragile X patients[6]. The Fragile X syndrome is related to the number of trinucleotide CGG repeats at the 5' untranslated region of the causative FMR-1 gene. Normal subjects have 6–50 CGG repeats. Carriers, referred to as premutation, 50–200 repeats. Affected individuals or full mutation have more than 200 repeats resulting in hypermethylation of the promoter region and repressed transcription of FMR-1[7].

Occurrence of the Fragile X Syndrome has been reported in Chinese but the prevalence is not known[8,9]. In one study in Taiwan it was the second commonest cause of chromosomal abnormality after Down's Syndrome in an institution of 341 mentally retarded children[10]. The number of reported occurrences of the disease in Mainland China and Taiwan suggests that its prevalence in Chinese is probably between 1 in 2000 and 1 in 4000. In this study we attempted to analyze the CGG repeat numbers in the Chinese population.

Materials and Methods

Subjects   Normal Chinese subjects were recruited in (a) Hong Kong: 497 voluntary staff and students in the Prince of Wales Hospital; (b) Shanghai: 50 students of the Shanghai Medical University; (c) Changsha: 40 members of the staff of the First Affiliated Hospital of the Hunan Medical University; (d) Dalian: 42 students of the Dalian Railway Medical College.

DNA Analysis   Genomic DNA was extracted from EDTA whole blood by a modification of the salting-out method[11]. Oligonucleotides were synthesized by GIBCO BRL (Gethersburg, MD, USA). For PCR the forward primer was the first 21 bp of the FMR-1 gene sequence (5'-GAC GGA GGC GCC GCT GCC AGG-3') and the backward primer the complement of FMR-1 152-132 (5'-GTG GGC TGC GGG CGC TCG AGG-3')[12]. The PCR procedure was modified from a described method[13]. Each PCR mixture contained 0.2 mmol/L each dATP, dCTP, dTTP and 7-deaza-2'-dGTP (Boehringer Mannheim, Mannheim, Germany), 0.75 mmol/L magnesium chloride, 10% dimethylsulfoxide, 60 ng forward primer, 40 ng backward primer, 100 ng DNA, 0.25 U *Taq* polymerase (GIBCO BRL) and 1 × PCR buffer (GIBCO BRL) to a final volume of 10 mL. After an initial denaturation at 94°C for 2 min, a 30-cycle PCR was carried out on a Perkin Elmer

Cetus thermal cycler: 94°C for 30 sec, 61°C for 1 min and 72°C for 2 min. The PCR products were electrophoresed on 6% polyacrylamide and blotted onto a Biodyne B positively charged nylon membrane (Biodyne B) on a semi-dry electroblotter (Hoefer Scientific Instruments, San Francisco, CA, USA). The amplified CCG repeats in the FMR-1 gene in the PCR products on the nylon were hybridized with a P^{32} labelled $(CGG)_5$ probe and detected by autoradiography. The CGG repeat number was calculated by matching with bands of pBR322 *Hpa*II ladder marker (GIBCO BRL).

Results

CGG repeat sizes in Chinese subjects in Hong Kong In 795 X chromosomes of 497 subjects (199 males and 298 females), 28 distinctly sized alleles were identified, ranging from 19 to 54 CGG repeats (Table 1). The most dominant repeat was 29, found in 298 of the 795 X chromosomes (37.5%), followed by 30 in 219 chromosomes (27.5%) and 31 in 88 chromosomes (11.1%). Over 76% of the chromosomes have one of these three size numbers. There was a minor peak at repeat 36 found in 69 chromosomes (8.7%). Only five chromosomes, 0.6% of the total, had alleles over 50 repeats, one with 52, three with 53 and one with 54.

CGG repeat sizes in Chinese female subjects in Hong Kong Among the female subjects, 98 were homozygotes and 200 heterozygotes, heterozygote frequency being 67.1% (Table 1). The most common homozygote was 29/29 in 53 subjects (17.8%) followed by 30/30 in 31 subjects (10.4%) and 31/31 in 8 subjects (2.7%). The combinations of the heterozygotes were very variable. Only one individual has both alleles below 20, who was a homozygote of 19/19. No one individual has both alleles greater than 40. There was a striking prominence of the commonest alleles, 29, 30 and 31. As many as 59% have these alleles only and only 6% of the subjects did not have any of them.

Comparison of CGG repeat patterns among subjects of different parts of China The patterns of CGG repeat sizes of individuals from the Chinese cities of Shanghai, Changsha and Dalian were similar to that of Hong Kong. The most common alleles were 29, 30 and 31. The spread of the repeats numbers was narrower presumably due to the smaller number of subjects. There was a variation in heterozygote frequencies, 54.1 for the Shanghai females, 77.3% for Changsha and 61.9% for Dalian. It is noted that the

Priscilla MK Poon, et al.

Table 1 Comparison of CGG repeat variation among normal subjects from different parts of China.

Number of CGG Repeats	Number of Alleles Observed (% age of Total)			
	Hong Kong 497 subjects 795 chromosomes	Shanghai 50 subjects 74 chromosomes	Changsha 40 subjects 62 chromosomes	Dalian 42 subjects 63 chromosomes
19	2 (0.3%)		1 (1.6%)	
20	1 (0.1%)			1 (1.6%)
22	2 (0.3%)			
23	3 (0.4%)	1 (1.4%)	1 (1.6%)	2 (3.2%)
24	2 (0.3%)	1 (1.4%)	1 (1.6%)	1 (1.6%)
25	3 (0.4%)		1 (1.6%)	1 (1.6%)
26	1 (0.1%)	1 (1.4%)		
28	5 (0.6%)			
29	298 (37.5%)	29 (39.2%)	25 (40.3%)	32 (50.8%)
30	219 (27.5%)	20 (27.0%)	14 (22.6%)	14 (22.2%)
31	88 (11.1%)	8 (10.8%)	6 (9.7%)	5 (7.9%)
32	31 (3.9%)	3 (4.1%)	1 (1.6%)	1 (1.6%)
34	4 (0.5%)			
35	4 (0.5%)			
37	69 (8.7%)	4 (5.4%)	6 (9.7%)	2 (3.2%)
37	15 (1.9%)			
38	3 (0.4%)			
39	7 (0.9%)			
40	7 (0.9%)			
41	5 (0.6%)			
42	1 (0.1%)			
43	4 (0.5%)			
44	2 (0.3%)			
45	1 (0.1%)			
52	1 (0.1%)			
53	3 (0.4%)		1 (1.6%)	
54	1 (0.1%)			

subjects from Dalian, which is the northernmost city, only have repeat sizes of 29, 30 and 31.

Discussion

In a population screening study, the number of CGG repeats in the FMR-1 gene in 309 unrelated X chromosomes in the Caucasians were found to be ranging from 13 to 49, most frequent allele at 29 repeats (22.5%). The secondary peak was at 19 and 22[14]. Similar distribution

Table 2 Allelic features of normal Chinese females

	Hong Kong	Shanghia	Changhsha	Dalian
Heterozygosity frequency	67%	54%	77%	61%
Total frequency of the homozygote 29/29, 30/30, 31/31	31%	46%	23%	28%
Total frequency of the heterozygote 29/30, 29/31, 30/31	28%	12%	32%	28%
Individuals only having the 29, 30 and 31 alleles	59%	58%	55%	76%
Individuals not having any 29, 30 or 31 alleles	6%	8%	13%	0%
individuals having a 36 alleles	15%	8%	18%	0%
Individuals not having any 29, 30, 31 or 36 alleles	2.3%	3%	4%	0%

Figure 1 Common CGG alleles observed in normal Chinese subjects. The CGG repeat sizes were calculated based on the molecular sizes of the labelled *Hpa*II digests of pBR322 in Lane M. Lanes a, e, f, g, h and i were males of repeat size 29, lane j a male with repeat 35. Lanes b and c were females heterozygous for 29/39, and lane d a female homozygous for 29/29.

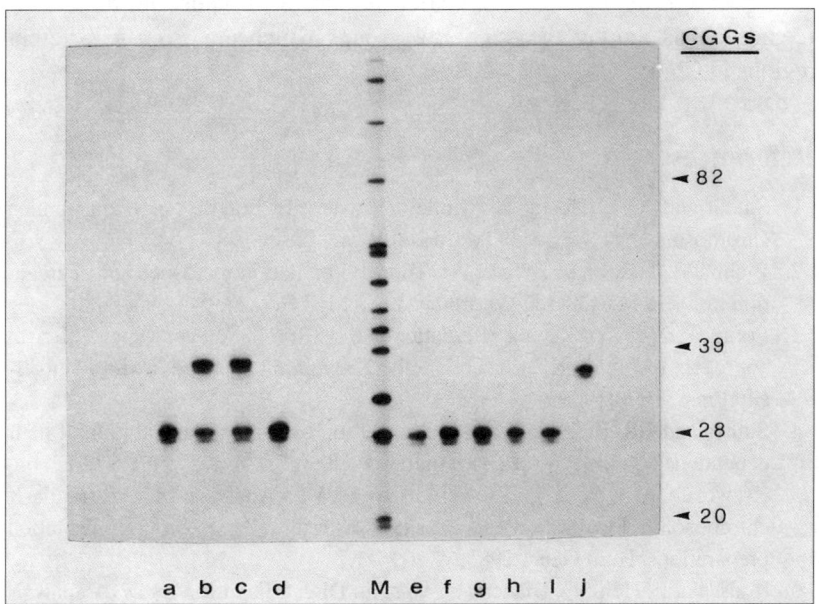

patterns were observed in the Spanish population based on PCR analysis of 208 normal chromosomes and the most frequent allele in a range of 18 to 54 repeats was 29 (24%)[15]. A new distribution pattern of the CGG repeat sizes was observed in 570 unrelated normal X chromosomes mostly from the white population with Caucasian background[13]. The most frequent allele was 30 (38.8%) with the secondary peaks at 20 and 23. The heterozygote frequency was 80%, which was higher than the 63% previously reported[12]. In a study of CGG repeats in Chinese the most frequent CGG allele was found to be 29 repeats[16]. There was no peak at either 19 or 22 repeats but a secondary peak appeared to be at 36. The overall heterozygote frequency was 70%.

In this study the distribution pattern of normal allele sizes among the X chromosomes in the Hong Kong population was found to be very similar to those from three different cities of China (Shanghai, Changsha and Dalian). All have the most frequent allele at 29 repeats and a secondary peak at 36 repeats. Our results suggest that a notable distribution pattern of CGG allele sizes, which is different from those observed in the Western populations, may exist in Chinese and that this pattern is relatively stable within the ethnic group. Meanwhile, the number of CGG repeats in the normal Chinese population is revealed in this study to be between 19 and 54 (Table 1). The "cut-off" point of a CGG repeat number of 54 in the normal subjects for Hans Chinese population is relevant because no major difference exists among the 4 control groups which are from 4 different regions in China.

References

1. Sutherland GR, Hecht F, Mulley JC, et al. Fragile sites on human chromosomes. New York: Oxford University Press, 1985.
2. Webb TP, Bundey SE, Thake AI, Todd J. Population incidence and segregation ratios in Martin-Bell syndrome. Am J Med Genet 1986;23:573–80.
3. Fryns JP. X-linked mental retardation and the fragile X syndrome: a clinical approach. In Davies KE, ed. The fragile X syndrome. Oxford: Oxford University Press, 1990:1–39.
4. Sutherland GR. Fragile sites on human chromosomes: demonstration of their dependence on the type of tissue culture medium. Science. 1977;197:265–6.
5. Krawczun MS, Jenkins EC and Brown WT. Analysis of the fragile-X chromosome: localisation and detection of the fragile site in high resolution preparations. Hum Genet 1985;69:209–11.
6. Rousseau F, Heitz D, Biancalana V, et al. Direct diagnosis by DNA analysis

of the fragile X syndrome of mental retardation. N Eng J Med 1991;325:1673–81.

7. Bell MV, Hirst MC, Nakahori Y, et al. Physical mapping across the fragile X: hypermethylation and clinical expression of the fragile X syndrome. Cell 1991;64:861–6.

8. Zhao Y, Shen Y, Liu Y, et al. Fragile X syndrome (Martin-Bell syndrome) in China. Am J Med Genet 1991;38:288–9.

9. Qin XB, Yang AD, Fei HB. The cytogenetic and clinical study of fragile X syndrome. Abstract 79, The International Conference on Molecular Biology of Genetic Diseases, Shanghai, China, 4–7 October 1992.

10. Li SY, Tsai CC, Chou MY, Lin JK. A cytogenetic study of mentally retarded school children in Taiwan with special reference to the fragile X chromosome. Hum Genet 1988;79:292–6.

11. Miller SA, Dykes DD, Polesky HF. A simple salting-out procedure for extracting DNA from human nucleated cells. Nucleic Acid Res 1988;16:1215.

12. Fu YH, Kuhl DPA, Pizzuti A, et al. Variation of the CGG repeat at the fragile X site results in genetic instablity: resolution of the Sherman paradox. Cell 1991;67:1047–58.

13. Brown WT, Houck GE Jr, Jeriorowsky A, et al. Rapid fragile X carrier screening and prenatal diagnosis using a nonradioactive PCR test. JAMA 1993;270:1569–75.

14. Jacobs PA, Bullman H, Macpherson J, et al. Population studies of the fragile X: a molecular approach. J Med Genet 1993;30:454–9.

15. Mila M, Kruyer H, Glover G, et.al. Molecular analysis of the (CGG)n expansion in the FMNR-1 gene in 59 Spanish fragile X syndrome families. Hum Genet 1994;94:395–400.

16. Zhong N, Liu X, Gou S, et al. Distribution of FMR-1 and associated microsatellite alleles in a normal Chinese population. Am J Med Genet 1994;51:417–22.

Rapid PCR Method for Fragile X Screening among Mentally Retarded Persons

Anita YY Ng, Stephen TS Lam*

*Clinical Genetic Service, Department of Health, Cheung Sha Wan Jockey Club Clinic, Shamshuipo, Kowloon, Hong Kong. * Corresponding author.*

Abstract *The fragile X syndrome is the most frequent form of inherited mental retardation and the most common chromosomal cause of mental retardation after trisomy 21. Therefore fragile X screening programme is essential. Since the phenotypic features occur irregularly among fragile X patients and mental retardation is almost always present, every mentally retarded patients without a known etiology must be screened for fragile X syndrome. However this constitutes a significant workload in many genetic laboratories. Since the great majority of these referrals will be negative, there is a need for a rapid and inexpensive screening test to screen for the presence of a normal allele by amplification across the CGG repeats (FRAXA) using polymerase chain reaction. FXD and FXE primers were used. 7-deaza-2'-deoxyguanosine triphosphate was incorporated in the PCR to destabilize secondary DNA structure and to allow successful amplification of GC rich segment (CGG repeats). Forty random samples from the mentally retarded persons were tested by this rapid PCR method and the conventional cytogenetic fragile X site induction method. Five patients were diagnosed to be fragile X males by both methods. The rapid PCR method showed that four patients could be either fragile X female or homozygous normal females. Further investigation by Southern blotting after EcoR1-Eagl digestion and StB12.3 probe should be conducted for confirmation of diagnosis.*

Introduction

In 1969, Herbert Lubs first reported the presence of a marker X chromosome in the form of a fragile site in a family in which nonspecific familial X-linked mental retardation was segregating. This constriction, or fragile site was observed near the terminal end of the long arm of the chromosome and was expressed in only a portion of the cells examined from a patient. Fragile X syndrome was the most frequent familial form of mental retardation in humans with an incidence of approximately 1 in 1250 males and 1 in 2000 females[1]. Next to trisomy 21, the fragile X syndrome was the most common specific chromosomal cause of mental retardation among mentally retarded boys. Although no clinical features could be considered pathognonomic for fragile X syndrome, some characteristics such as marcroorchidism, prognathism, large protuberant ears, and a high-arched palate had been consistently documented and were clinically significant[2]. Mental retardation was the major phenotypic consequence of inheriting the fragile X locus and both sexes might be affected, although males were typically more severe[3]. Clinical diagnosis was often difficult, particularly in females, and had in the past relied heavily upon the cytogenetic demonstration of the fragile site at Xq27.3 which was associated with the syndrome[4]. Recently the Fragile X Mental Retardation-1 (FMR1) gene at the fragile X locus had been identified and cloned[5]. Two molecular differences of the FMR-1 gene had been found in fragile X patients: a size increase of an FMR-1 exon containing a CGG repeat and abnormal methylation of a CpG island 250 bp proximal to this repeat[6]. These molecular characteristics had greatly enhanced the identification of affected individuals and carriers of the population who were not detected cytogenetically. Present data on X-linked mental retardation confirmed that fragile X screening by cytogenetic studies was positive in no more than 40–50 per cent of the males with X-linked mental retardation. Many experienced laboratories now routinely conduct a fragile X analysis (either cytogenetic or molecular) on all specimens, male and female, referred for mental retardation of unknown etiology or simply for developmental delay. This had been surprisingly fruitful in ascertaining fragile X males and females and should be encouraged as a standard of molecular and cytogenetic practice[3]. However, since this practice would greatly increase the workload of the laboratories, a rapid screening method which allowed amplification of the triplet CGG repeat sequence at the FRAXA locus by polymerase chain reaction (PCR) and detection of the products on non-denaturing gels stained with ethidium bromide would be very cost-effective[7]. In this way, alleles of normal size would be detected, leaving a small minority of samples to be tested by Southern blotting involving the use of double digestion (EcoRI and Eagl) and StB12.3 probe[6].

Objectives

Firstly a rapid PCR method using FXD and FXE primers which amplify across the CGG repeats of the FRAXA alleles was set up. 7-deaza-2'-deoxyguanosine triphosphate is incorporated in the PCR. Secondly the effectiveness of this PCR method was compared with the cytogenetic fragile X site induction method. Forty blood samples from forty different mentally retarded patients are tested with both methods.

Materials and Methods

Cytogenetic Analysis   Heparin blood samples are cultured 3 days in folate/thymidine deficient system[8], were then harvested and stained with Leishman for fragile X site detection. For males 100 cells were analyzed and for females 150.

PCR Analysis   DNA was isolated by phenol-chloroform extraction. 100ng DNA sample was mixed with 200ng each of primer FXD (5' TGA CGG AGG CGC CGC TGC CAG GGG GCG TGG3')and primer FXE (5'GAG AGG TGG GCT GCG GGC GCT CGT CGA GGC CCA3') for the amplification of the CGG repeat of FRAXA, 200ng each of primer ARA (5' ACC AGG TAG CCT GTG GGG CCT CTA CGA TGG 3') and primer ARC (5'CCA GAA GCC GCG AGC GCA GCA C3') for the amplification of the CAG repeat of the coding region of the androgen receptor gene in X-linked Spinal Bulbar Muscular Atrophy (internal control for inhibitors in DNA preparation), 200μmol/L each of dATP, dCTP and dTTP, 150μ mol/L dGTP, 50μ mol/L 7-deaza-2'dGTP, 10% dimethysulphoxide in a total volume of 50μl containing Taq Polymerase Buffer (33.5mM Tris-HCl (pH8.8), 8.3mM $(NH_4)_2SO_4$, 1mM Mg Cl_2 and 85ug/ml Bovine Serum Albumin). After denaturation of the PCR reaction mix at 95°C for 10 min, 2.5U of Taq DNA Polymerase was added while maintains the temperature at 95°C. It was then subjected to 30 cycles of amplification: 95°C for 1 min; 64°C for 1.5 min; 72°C for 2 min with a final extension of 5 min at 72°C[7]. Ten ul of PCR product was analyzed by electrophoresis in 2% agarose gel containing 3ul ethidium bromide. The presence of two bands in the correct size range (86-224bp for FRAXA allele and 294-321bp for AR allele) in a male, or heterozygosity for alleles of normal size in a female, exclude the presence of an expansion mutation at either the FRAXA or the AR locus. In order to detect females who were heterozygous for normal alleles at the FRAXA locus, improved resolution was obtained on a 20 cm

8% nondenaturing polyacrylalmide gel by electrophoresis for 14 hours at 160V in $1 \times$ TBE[9].

Results

Results of the rapid polymerase chain reaction and cytogenetic diagnosis of the 40 samples are summarized as follows:

Sample No.	Fragile X site (% FRAXQ27.3)	Polymerase Chain Reaction	
		2% agarose gel	8% nondenaturing polyacrylamide gel
1.	0	normal male	
2.	0	heterozygous normal female	
3.	0	normal male	
4.	0	$\Rightarrow$	heterozygous normal female
5.	0	normal male	
6.	0	normal male	
7.	0	normal male	
8.	0	normal male	
9.	0	$\Rightarrow$	heterozygous normal female
10.	0	normal male	
11.	0	normal male	
12.	0	$\Rightarrow$	heterozygous normal female/ fragile X female
13.	0	$\Rightarrow$	heterozygous normal female
14.	0	normal male	
15.	0	normal male	
16.	12	fragile X male	
17.	0	normal male	
18.	0	normal male	
19.	0	$\Rightarrow$	heterozygous normal female/ fragile X female
20.	0	$\Rightarrow$	heterozygous normal female/ fragile X female
21.	0	$\Rightarrow$	heterozygous normal female
22.	4	fragile X male	
23.	0	$\Rightarrow$	fragile X female
24.	19	fragile X male	
25.	0	normal male	
26.	0	normal male	
27.	0	normal male	
28.	16	fragile X male	
29.	0	heterozygous normal female	
30.	0	normal male	
31.	0	normal male	
32.	0	normal male	

Sample No.	Fragile X site (% FRAXQ27.3)	Polymerase Chain Reaction	
		2% agarose gel	8% nondenaturing polyacrylamide gel
33.	0	normal male	
34.	0	normal male	
35.	0	normal male	
36.	0	normal male	
37.	0	normal male	
38.	0	normal male	
39.	16	fragile X male	
40.	0	normal male	

Figure 1   Sample 16 showed a fragile site at Xq27.3.

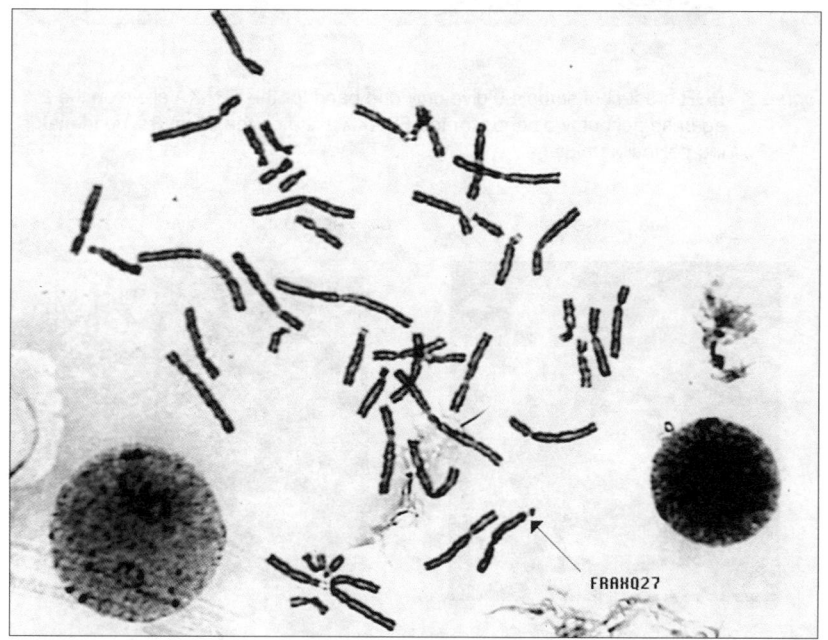

Figure 2   G-banding of the same metaphase. To confirm the chromosome's identity
(Sample 16)

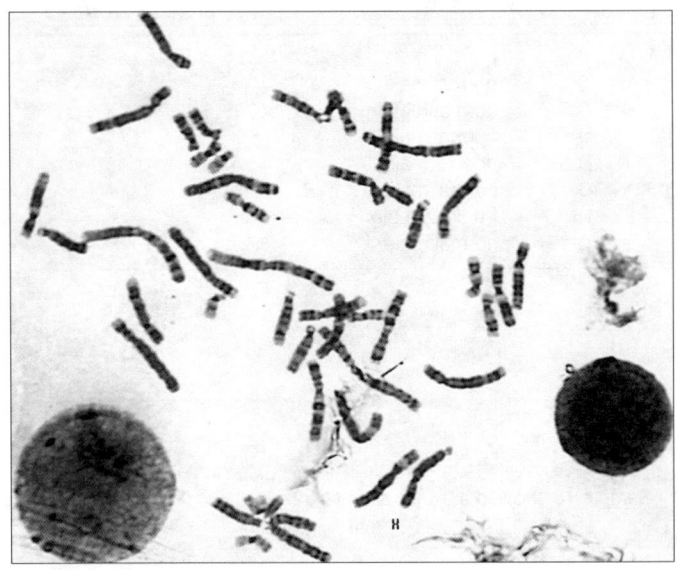

Figure 3   PCR product of sample 9 give only one band for the FRAXA allele on the 2%
agarose gel but two bands for the FRAXA allele on the 20cm 8% nondenaturing polyacrylamide gel.

2% agarose gel   8% nondenaturing polyacrylmide gel

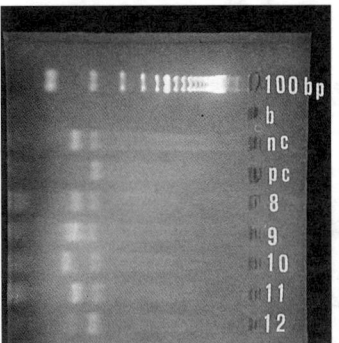
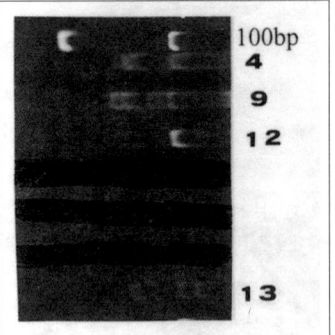

100bp   100bse pair ladder
nc   normal male control
pc   fragile X male control
b   blank (PCR conditions without DNA)

Discussion

Cytogenetic Analysis One hundred and fifty metaphases were analyzed for female subjects because detection of the fragile X site is more difficult and frequencies of expression are lower in females than in males. If the positive rate is less than 4%, the analysis would be repeated to confirm the diagnosis to exclude any artifacts. The presence of Xq27.3 fragile site must be confirmed with chromosome banding (Figure 1& 2). This is essential to distinguish the fragile X site definitely from the constitutive fragile site on chromosome 6 & 7, as well as the recently described folate-sensitive constitutive site in the X-chromosome at Xq27.2 that is clearly distant from the Xq27.3 which is the fragile X syndrome site[10]. Among the 40 samples analyzed, five of them (Sample 16, 22, 24, 28 & 39) were found to have Xq27.3 fragile site.

Polymerase Chain Reaction Analysis The fragile site at Xq27.3 FRAXA is caused by expansion of an unstable CGG repeat at the 5' end of the FMR1 gene[5]. The two primers FXD and FXE are the two primers which flank the CGG repeat for the amplification. The presence of a high G+C content in the target DNA presents difficulties for in vitro DNA amplification across CG rich triplet repeats. On occasions, either a given pair of primers yields a high background of non-specific products, including primer-dimer artifacts and a low yield of the desired product, or there is no apparent amplification of the desired product. In this experiment the G+C content in the FRAXA fragment is between 81% (2CGG repeats) and 93% (52 CGG repeats). The incorporation of 7-deaza-2'-deoxyguanosine triphosphate (C^7dGTP) is to destabilize secondary DNA structure allows successful amplification of GC rich segment11. Taq DNA polymerase incorporates C^7dGTP with kinetics similar to those of dGTP incorporation[12]. Because the N-7 position of the guanine ring is replaced with a methine moiety[13], 7-deazaguanine precludes Hoogsteen bond formation (stacking) without affecting Watson-Crick base pairing. PCR products with a high content of C^7dGTP do not stain efficiently with ethidium bromide[14], presumably because adjacent base stacking is diminished in the C^7dGTP containing DNA. A ratio of 1:3 (1 C^7dGTP : 3 dGTP) is found to allow amplification of FRAXA alleles within the normal range (6-52 CGG repeats) and efficient staining of the PCR products with ethidium bromide.

Internal control primers ARC and ARD are incorporated to co-amplify the androgen receptor gene with FMR1 as a measure of inhibitors in the DNA preparation[15]. The largest FRAXA allele amplified by this protocol contained 53 repeats (as measured by a radioactive PCR assay and sized on a sequencing gel[16]). Thus normal male sample will give a single band on the agarose gel at the correct, normal size (86bp for 6 CGG repeats to 224bp for 52 CGG repeats). In contrast, male with full mutations and premutations give no visible bands.

Among the 40 samples analyzed, 5 samples (sample 16, 4, 24, 8 & 39) show no visible band for FRAXA locus. These are male samples and their PCR results indicated that they are fragile X male and this result coincides with the cytogenetic fragile X site findings. Thus this PCR methods is very useful for diagnosing male patients.

Female contains two X chromosome, female in which two FRAXA alleles of normal size are detected on 2% agarose gel can be scored as normal for FRAXA. An allele with a premutation or a full mutation will not be amplified by this PCR techniques due to the high G+C content and only one band is obtained. However the possibilities that the female sample is from a normal homozygous female cannot be ruled out. It is because the two FRAXA alleles may be of the same size and they coincide to give one single band only. Sample 2 & 29 are detected to be heterozygous with the resolving power of the minigel (2% agarose gel). To detect females who are heterozygous for normal alleles at the FRAXA locus, improved resolution can be obtained by running the same PCR product on a 20cm non denaturing 8% polyacrylamide gel (Figure 3). Sample 4, 9, 13 & 21 showed only one band in the 2% agarose gel however two normal bands are obtained in the polyacrylamide gel. Indicating that they are heterozygous normal females.

Sample 12 19 20 & 23 give only one band for the FRAXA allele on both the 2% agarose gel or the 8% non-denaturing polyacryalmide gel indicating that they may be homozygous females with normal alleles or fragile X females. Further investigation such as methylation detection using double digestion with both EcoRI & Eagl restriction enzymes and StB12.3 hybridization probe is required[6]. Sample 23 is highly suspected to be a fragile X female as her two brothers, sample 22 & 24, are confirmed to be fragile X males. The cytogenetic method takes fifteen working days to perform 40 samples whereas the PCR method take less than five working days to perform 40 samples.

Conclusion

The incorporation of the C^7dGTP in the PCR allows successful amplification of CGG repeats and efficient staining of the PCR products with ethidium bromide. PCR method is more rapid than the cytogenetic method and thus a better screening test. It is also more informative than the cytogenetic method. Four patients were shown to be potentially either fragile X female or homozygous normal females. Further investigation such as Southern Blotting techniques with double enzyme (EcoRI-Eagl) digestion and hybridization with StB12.3 probe should be conducted to confirm the expansion of the FMR-1 gene in these patients.

References

1. Webb TP, Bundey SE, Thake AI, Todd J. Population incidence and segregation ratios in the Martin-Bell syndrome. Am J Med Genet 1986; 23:537–80.
2. Martin JP, Bell J. A pedigree of mental defect showing sex-linkage. J Neuro Psychi 1943;6:154–7.
3. Barch MJ. The Act Cytogenetics Laboratory manual, 2nd ed. New York: Raven Press, 1991:493–5.
4. Sutcliff JS, Nelsen DL, Zhang F, et al. DNA methylation represses FMR1 transcription in fragile X syndrome. Hum Mol Genet 1992;1:400.
5. Verkerk AJMH, Pieretti M, Sutcliffe JS, et al. Identification of a gene (FMR1) containing a CGG repeat coincident with a breakpoint cluster region exhibiting length variation in fragile X syndrome. Cell 1991;65:905–14.
6. Oberle I, Rousseau F, Heitz D, et al. Instability of a 550 base pair DNA segment and abnormal methylation in fragile X syndrome. Science 1991; 252:1097–102.
7. Wang Q, Green E, Bobrow M, Matthew CG. A rapid, non-radioactive screening test for fragile X mutations at the FRAXA and FRAXE loci. J Med Genet 1995;32:170–3.
8. Jacky PB, Ahuja YR, Anyane-Yeboa K, et al. Guidelines for the preparation and analysis of the fragile X chromosome in lymphocytes. Am J Med Genet 1991;38:400–3.
9. Sambrook J, Fritsch EF, Maniatis T. Molecular cloning — a laboratory manual. 2nd ed. USA: Cold Spring Harbor Laboratory Press, 1992.
10. Sutherland GR, Baker E. Characterization of a new rare fragile site easily confused with the fragile X. Hum Mol Genet 1992;1:111–3.
11. Innis MA. PCR with 7-deaza-2'-deoxyguanosine triphosphate, in PCR protocols: a guide to methods and application. California: Academic Press, 1990:54–9.
12. Innis MA, Myambo KB, Gelfand DH, Brow MAD. DNA sequencing with thermus aquaticus DNA polymerase and direct sequencing of polymerase

chain reaction-amplified DNA. Proc Natl Acad Sci USA 1988;85:9436–40.

13. Barr P J, Thayer RM, Laybourn P, et al. 7-Deaza-2'-deoxyguanosine-5'-triphosphate; enhanced resolution in M13 dideoxy sequencing. Bio-Techniques 1988;4:428–32.

14. Latimer LJP, Lee JS. Ethidium bromide does not fluorescence when intercalated adjacent to 7-deazaguanine in duplex DNA. J Bio Chem 1991;266:13849–51.

15. Fu WH, Kuhl DPA, Pizzuti A, et al. Variation of the CGG repeat at the Fragile X site results in genetic instability — resolution of the Sherman Paradox. Cell 1991;76:1047–58.

16. Wang Q, Green E, Barnicoat A, et al. Cytogenetic versus DNA diagnosis in routine referrals for fragile X syndrome. Lancet 1993;342:1025–6.

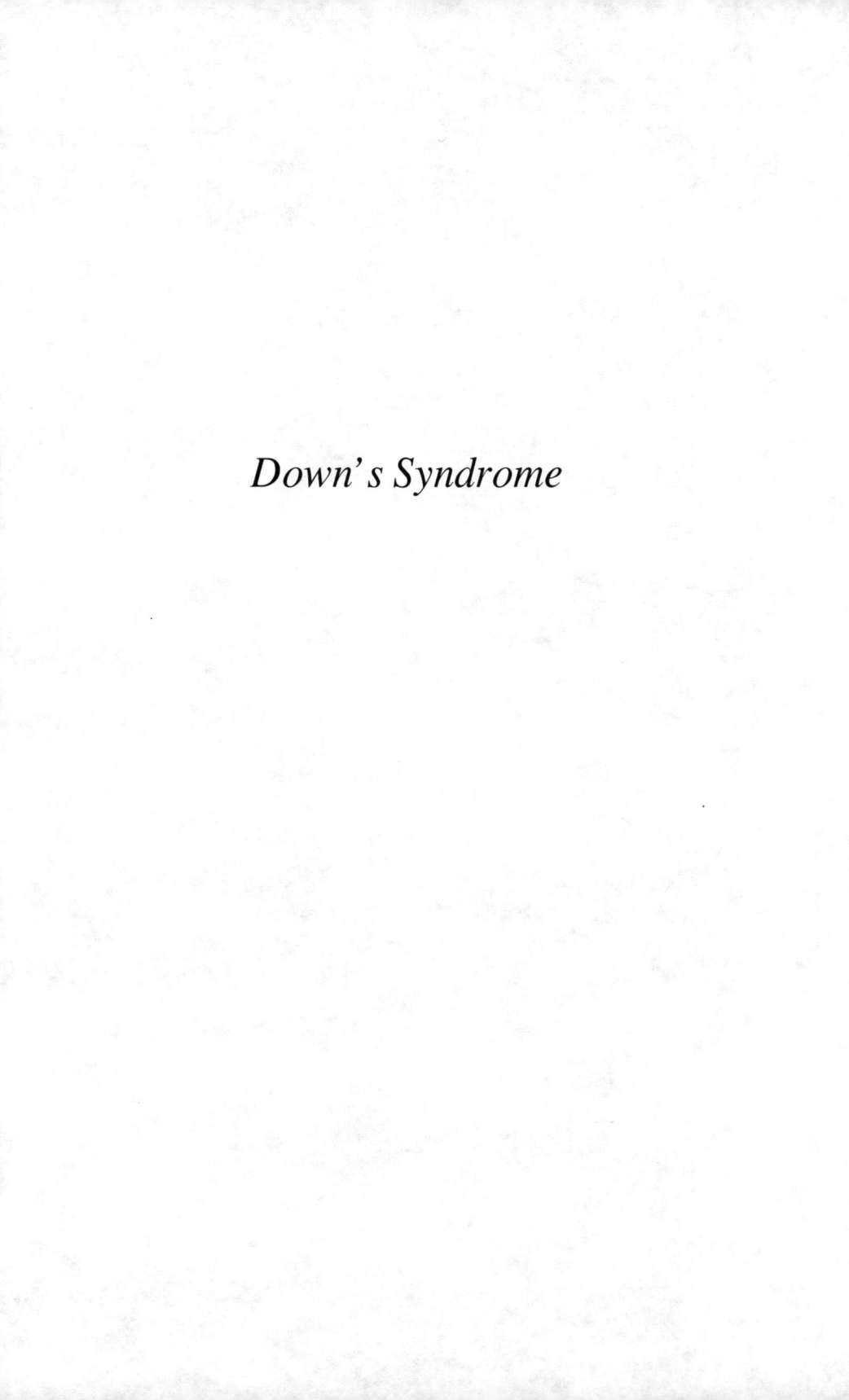

Down's Syndrome

Introduction of Maternal Serum Screening to Auckland, New Zealand

D Webster[2,3]*, J Dixon J[1], D Dixon-McIver[2], J France[3], J Giles[2,3], G Jackson[4], B Knox[2], A Roberts[2,3], R Ryall[5], I Winship[2,3]

[1] Capital Coast Health, Wellington, NZ. [2] Auckland Healthcare, Auckland, NZ. [3] University of Auckland, Auckland, NZ. [4] North Health, Auckland, NZ. [5] Department of Chemical Pathology, Women's and Children's Hospital, Adelaide, Australia. * Corresponding author.

Abstract We report the introduction of a pilot maternal serum screening programme to Auckland, New Zealand. The programme uses the chemistry and algorithm previously used in South Australia (SAMSAS) to screen for neural tube defects and chromosome abnormalities (primarily Down Syndrome). In order to address potential problems identified from the literature an information sheet for women was developed; the screening is offered only by practitioners who have attended a provider training course. Signed informed consent is required with all samples. Follow-up is co-ordinated by a genetic counsellor and mostly occurs at one hospital. The normal population established in South Australia was used. Assay comparability was established by use of identical technology and the analysis of 200 patient samples. Control materials supplied by SAMSAS are used in all assays. Results are reported as increased risk or low risk for chromosome abnormalities (1:50 and 1:2700) and neural tube defects (1:130 and 1:2500). Early results (400 patients screened) show a recall rate of 2.5% for neural tube defects and 11.5% for chromosome abnormalities. Adjusted for incorrect gestational age recall rates are 2.5% and 10.8%. The average age of our screened population is 31.7 years and the unadjusted recall rate from SAMSAS for 32 year old women is 8.53%. In addition to screening an older population, we are screening a population ethnically and socioeconomically atypical of the Auckland population. There may also be a higher incidence of "at-risk" pregnancies than are found in the normal population.

Introduction

We report the introduction of a pilot maternal serum screening programme to Auckland, New Zealand. There is no history of maternal blood testing for congenital abnormalities in New Zealand and the uptake of screening for Down syndrome using maternal age as the indicator for a diagnostic test is about 50%. The programme uses the chemistry and algorithm previously reported as used in South Australia (SAMSAS) to screen for neural tube defects and chromosome abnormalities (primarily Down Syndrome). We are confident that the laboratory aspects of the screening will be successful, and the main aim of the pilot programme is to assess whether the screening is acceptable to the community and what the likely costs of a full programme (additional cytogenetics, genetic counselling, ultrasounds) will be.

Methods

Maternal serum screening programmes in other countries have identified a number of problems caused by the screening, primarily that women have been unaware of the implications of the test they were having or of the risk meaning of the test results and secondarily that the diagnostic and counselling services are sometimes not well co-ordinated. In order to address these potential problems in a new screening programme, an information sheet for women was developed; the screening is offered only by practitioners who have attended a provider training course and received a comprehensive set of resource material about the screening; signed informed consent is required with all samples and follow-up is co-ordinated by a genetic counsellor and mostly occurs at one hospital. A genetic counsellor is available to women at all stages of screening. The Down Syndrome Association and Spina Bifida support group contribute to the provider education and offer telephone counselling to women. Providers were asked to offer the test to all women presenting for maternity care earlier than 16 weeks gestation.

Results and Discussion

Screening has been accepted by 92% of the women to whom it is offered. This is somewhat higher than might be expected from the literature and indicates that complete records of women refusing the test are not being kept or that the screening is being offered mostly to women who are likely to accept the test. Informal discussion with providers suggests that the latter is the case.

The normal population established in South Australia was used. Assay comparability was established by use of identical technology and the analysis of 200 patient samples. Control materials supplied by SAMSAS are used in all assays and other material in most assays.

Results are reported as increased risk or low risk for chromosome abnormalities (1:50 and 1:2700) and neural tube defects (1:130 and 1:2500). The risk results are empirical and derived from the South Australian experience.

Early results (800 patients screened) show a recall rate of 2.5% for neural tube defects and 10.3% for chromosome abnormalities. Adjusted for incorrect gestational age recall rates are 2.5% and 9.6%. The average age of our screened population is 31.7 years and the average age of women giving birth at our hospital is 28.2 years. The unadjusted recall rate from SAMSAS for 32 year old women is 8.53%. Thus the older age of our screened population accounts for almost all the increased recall rate. In addition to screening an older population, we are screening a population ethnically and socioeconomically atypical of the Auckland population. There may also be a higher incidence of "at-risk" pregnancies than are found in the normal population since a greater proportion of screened women come from specialist obstetric care or special hospital clinics than the women delivering at this hospital.

The screening programme in the Northern Region of the UK has some selective screening and some population screening. The recall rate for Down syndrome screening is 3.8% in population screening units and 10.2% in selective screening units (J Burn, personal communication).

The uptake of amniocentesis following an increased risk result on the Down syndrome screen may be used as an indicator of how well women understood the implications of the test (although some women will have changed their mind about the test in the time between taking the test and getting the result). 84 of the 88 women offered amniocentesis have accepted, showing the pretest counselling is effective. A client questionnaire is planned to more specifically address this question.

To-date (this data is clearly preliminary as most of the pregnancies screened have not yet come to term) the programme has identified 2 neural tube defects (one major spinal lesion, one anencephaly); 2 unsuspected sets of twins with increased risk NTD results (2 sets of twins had low-risk NTD results); 2 chromosome abnormalities coincident with increased risk Down syndrome screen results (XXY and XXX with an inversion); 2 unsuspected fetal deaths and a case of X-linked icthyosis (steroid sulphatase deficiency).

The programme continues as a pilot until June 30 1996. It is likely that because of the atypical, selected nature of our screened population we will not be able to fully answer the questions the pilot programme was designed to; it may be the pilot will need to continue until some population screening data are available.

Organization of a Biochemical Screening Programme for Down's Syndrome at Kwong Wah Hospital, Hong Kong

Connie OS Yuen*, SY Sin, A Ghosh, Lawrence CH Tang

*Department of Obstetrics and Gynaecology, Kwong Wah Hospital, Kowloon, Hong Kong. * Corresponding author.*

Abstract *A voluntary screening programme for Down's syndrome using maternal serum alpha-fetoprotein (AFP) and human chorionic gonadotrophin (hCG) measurements was carried out at Kwong Wah Hospital. All women aged <35 and with gestation age <18 weeks were given information pamphlets about the programme. Individual counselling, verbal consent and dating ultrasound scan were performed at the first antenatal visit. Maternal serum samples for AFP and hCG were arranged at 16–18 weeks of gestation. If the Down's syndrome risk was ≥1:250, the couple would be counselled and offered amniocentesis. Subsequent management plan depended on the karyotype and parental choice. From September 1994 to April 1995, 979 pregnant women were recruited, 765 (78%) consented for screening and 761 serum samples were obtained. 12 (1.6%) were screened positive and all had amniocentesis with normal karyotype. Our experience confirms that implementation of a Down's screening programme requires the provision of information and expert counselling services to clients, laboratory support, ultrasound examination and amniocentesis, and adequate after-care or grief counselling if the pregnancy is terminated. Health-care providers must not overlook the high level of parental anxiety involved during the screening process.*

Introduction

Down's Syndrome is one of the commonest causes of severe mental retardation. The overall incidence in our local population in Hong Kong is 1:1100. The risk of fetal Down's Syndrome increases with advancing maternal age. The current practice in Kwong Wah Hospital is to offer amniocentesis or chorionic villus sampling to women aged 35 and above to screen for Down's Syndrome. Using the maternal age alone as the screening test , 30% of the Down's Syndrome babies will be detected theoretically since only 12% of the mothers over 35 years of age are currently undergoing amniocentesis. The majority of infants with Down's Syndrome are born among women younger than age 35, as they account for about 90% of all pregnancies. Pregnancies affected by Down's Syndrome have lower levels of maternal serum alphafetoprotein (AFP), elevated levels of maternal serum chorionic gonadotrophin (hCG), and lower levels of maternal serum oestriol (E3). The dual test, using AFP and hCG but not oestriol, has a detection rate of around 60% and a false positive rate of 3.5–6.3%. Inclusion of oestriol adds little advantage to the detection rate, but will increase the false positive rate and the cost. We have conducted a screening programme in our hospital by measuring AFP and hCG.

Methods

Screening for Down's Syndrome using AFP and hCG was started in Kwong Wah Hospital (KWH) with the Department of Obstetrics and Gynaecology of the University of Hong Kong in September 1994. Screen positive was defined as a calculated risk of equal to or greater than 1:250. This should result in the detection of 55–60% of fetal Down's Syndrome, in which 40% would not be detected by this screening test.

In our screening programme at KWH all women younger than age 35 and before 18 weeks of gestation will be given information pamphlets on the biochemical screening programme and explanation of the protocol when attending booking session. After obtaining verbal consent, individual counselling and dating scan will be performed at the first antenatal visit. Maternal serum samples for AFP and hCG will be arranged at 16–18 weeks of gestation and sent to the laboratory at Tsan Yuk Hospital for analysis. If the Down's Syndrome risk is 1:250 or above, the couple would be counselled and offered amniocentesis. Subsequent management plan depends on the karyotype and parental choice.

Results

From September 1994 to April 1995, the total number of women attending our booking sessions was 2798. Of these 979 patients were recruited. 765(78%) consented for screening and 721 blood samples were obtained for serum analysis. 12 were screened positive and all had amniocentesis with normal karyotype. 12 had raised AFP and 2 with low hCG. Fetal abnormalities detected included anencephaly(2), omphalocele(1) and 47XXY(1).

Practical issues encountered.

During the implementation and execution of our screening programme, we have encountered a number of issues which should have been dealt with:

(1) Staff education.
(2) Laboratory services with split site problem-serum samples from KWH to TYH.
(3) Counselling to women on: Down's Syndrome programme, definitive diagnosis if screen positive, fetus diagnosed to have Down's Syndrome, option of termination or continuation of pregnancy and future prognosis; ultrasound services and loading of antenatal clinic.
(4) Wrong data on prenatal biochemical screening assay request form.
(5) Quality control and efficiency of the programme.

Conclusions

Our preliminary experience confirms that the implementation of a Down's Syndrome Programme requires the provision of information and counselling services to clients, access to expert advice and laboratory support, efficient ultrasound examination and amniocentesis, and adequate after care or grief counselling if the pregnancy is terminated. Health care providers must not overlook the high level of parental anxiety involved during the screening process. Pilot study of prenatal biochemical screening programme can be implemented in any services unit provided that resources for staff education and patient counselling, provision of ultrasound, genetic and obstetric facilities are available.

Biochemical Screening in the Prince of Wales Hospital, Hong Kong

Hedy YM Fung[1]*, Michael S Rogers[1], Tze Kin Lau[1], [2]Eric LK Law, [2]M Hjelm

[1] Department of Obstetrics & Gynaecology, The Chinese University of Hong Kong, Shatin, Hong Kong. [2] Department of Chemical Pathology, The Chinese University of Hong Kong, Shatin, Hong Kong. * Corresponding author.

Abstract *Significantly lower incidence of trisomy 21 has been observed in the older Chinese women in the Prince of Wales Hospital, Hong Kong, than was expected when compared with indigenous Europeans. Biochemical screening for trisomy 21 in the younger age group of pregnant women would in theory be more cost effective for the detection of trisomy 21. A preliminary study was performed on 193 Chinese pregnant women with singleton pregnancy between 14 and 21 weeks of gestation. The results of the regressed median levels of AFP and HCG were compared with the Taiwan Chinese data which was based on 500 pregnant women in each week of the gestation. There were 362 Chinese pregnant women with singleton pregnancy that had undergone biochemical screening for Down's syndrome between 7th August and 31st October 1995. The results of the two maternal serum markers were compared with the results of the preliminary study as well as the Taiwan Chinese data base. Among the 193 pregnant women in the preliminary study, 14.0% were of age 35 or over. The rate of positive results for Down's syndrome was 7.8%, of which 46.7% were from pregnant women younger than 35. All babies were normal at delivery. Among the 362 pregnant women, 10.5% were of age 35 or over. The rate of positive results was 0.8% of which 33.3% were from pregnant women younger than 35. All 3 pregnant women had normal fetal karyotyping. The difference in the initial positive rate for Down's syndrome between the preliminary study and the service period may be due to the different distribution of older pregnant women of age 35 or above and the more stringent ultrasound scanning and calculation of gestational age employed during the service period.*

Introduction

Significantly lower incidence of trisomy 21 was previously observed in older pregnant women in Asian immigrants in Europe when compared with indigenous Europeans[1]. A retrospective study on the age-related incidence of trisomy 21 in Chinese pregnant women over a nine-year period in the Prince of Wales Hospital, Hong Kong, has shown a similar pattern of results. Biochemical screening for trisomy 21 in the younger age group of pregnant women in theory would therefore be more cost-effective in detection of trisomy 21.

Subjects and Methods

Preliminary Study   Among women who attended the Prince of Wales Hospital for antenatal care between August 1993 and March 1994, 193 Chinese pregnant women with singleton pregnancy between the gestations of 14 and 21 weeks without Down's syndrome or neural tube defect had screening test for Down's syndrome using two serum markers, alpha-fetaoprotein (AFP) and human chorionic gonadotrophin (HCG). All had ultrasound scan for confirmation of the gestation. The ultrasound scan was performed by the obstetricians who saw the women in the antenatal clinic. Gestational age calculated from the last menstrual period was accepted if the biparietal diameter was within $\pm$ 2SD for the gestation. Maternal weight measurement was available in all pregnant women.

The regressed median levels of AFP and HCG of these 193 pregnant women were compared with the data of a study on Taiwan Chinese, which involved 500 pregnant women in each week of the gestation between 15 to 21 weeks.

Biochemical Screening Service   Between 7th August and 31st October 1995, biochemical screening test using two markers were performed on 362 Chinese pregnant women attending Prince of Wales Hospital. All pregnant women had singleton pregnancy and were between 15 to 20 weeks of gestation. The gestation was calculated from the combined measurements of biparietal diameter, head circumference, abdominal circumference and femur length using the formula provided by the ultrasound machine (Acuson 128PX). The scan was performed only by three obstetricians to minimize inter-observer variation. Maternal weight was obtained at the time of the test.

Maternal serum AFP and HCG were measured by Microparticle

Enzyme Immunoassay (MEIA) on the Abbott Imx immunoassay analyzer (Abbott Laboratories, U.S.A.). The risk estimates for Down's syndrome were derived by a complex mathematical calculation that combines the maternal serum markers concentrations with the prior odds of a Down's syndrome fetus based on maternal age. The calculation was performed using an AFP/Sample Management Software Plus (Robert Maciel Associates Inc.). The software utilizes the Wald model[2].

Results

Preliminary Study   The preliminary study on the regressed median levels of AFP and HCG between 14 and 21 weeks of gestation in our local population showed comparable results to the Taiwan Chinese data. Among the 193 pregnant women, 27 (14.0%) were of age 35 or over. There were 15 cases (7.8%) positive for Down's syndrome (risk ≥ 1/270) in the preliminary study. Seven (46.7%) of these were from pregnant women younger than age 35. Clinical examination showed that all babies were normal at delivery.

Biochemical Screening Service   Biochemical screening for Down's syndrome between 15 and 20 weeks of gestation has been commenced since 7th August 1995 in the Prince of Wales Hospital.

Between 7th August and 31st October 1995, there were 362 biochemical screening tests performed. Among these 362 pregnant women, 38 (10.5%) were of age 35 or over. Three cases (0.8%) were considered high risk for Down's syndrome. One (33.3%) of these was from a pregnant woman younger than age 35. All 3 pregnant women underwent amniocentesis for chromsomal studies after counselling. Normal fetal karyotyping was obtained in all cases.

We undertook repeated statistical comparison between the results of this group of pregnant women and the results obtained from our preliminary study. Similar analysis was also applied to the Taiwan Chinese data at various stages. Our results revealed no significant difference in the median levels of the two serum markers. As a result, the new median levels of the two markers have been constantly revised accordingly.

Discussion

Despite no significant difference in the median levels of the two serum markers was obtained between the three groups of results, there was a difference in the initial positive rate for Down's syndrome between the preliminary study and the first phase of the service period. The difference may be partly accounted for by the distribution of older pregnant women of age 35 or over, 14.0% of the total study subjects in the preliminary study belonged to this group of women compared with only 10.5% in the service period.

The other possible reason for the discrepancy may be due to the employment of more stringent conditions for ultrasound scanning and calculation of gestational age during the service period. The effect of reliable ultrasound scan determination of gestational age on the screening performance of the biochemical screening test has already been confirmed[3]. The aim of using combined measurements of biparietal diameter, head circumference, abdominal circumference, femur length and using the same formula provided by ultrasound machine for calculation of gestational age is to provide a more uniform and objective basis for accurate assessment of the risk of Down's syndrome. The results obtained would form a reliable data base.

The number of cases during the initial phase of the service period is small. More definite and clearer conclusions could be drawn when more information are accumulated in future.

References

1. Rogers MS. Racial variations in the incidence of trisomy 21. Br J Obstet Gynaecol 1986;93:597–9.
2. Wald NJ, Cuckle HS, Densem JW, et al. Maternal serum screening for Down Syndrome in early pregnancy. Br Med J 1988;297:883–7.
3. Wald NJ, Cuckle HS, Densem JW, Kennard A, Smith D. Maternal serum screening for Down's syndrome: the effect of routine ultrasound scan deter-mination of gestational age and adjustment for maternal weight. Br J Obstet Gynaecol 1992;99:144–9.

Congenital Hypothyroidism

Value of Very Early Repeat TSH Determination in Newborns with Elevated Cord Serum TSH Levels

Roy Joseph*, Kim Leong Tan

*Department of Paediatrics, National University of Singapore, National University Hospital, 5 Lower Kent Ridge Road, Singapore 0511. * Corresponding author.*

Abstract   *Cord serum TSH screening for congenital hypothyroidism has the disadvantage of a high recall rate of about 1%. We investigated the usefulness of measuring the TSH levels (mU/L) as soon as being informed of an elevated cord level. From June 1994 to October 1995, 4706 newborns had cord serum TSH (TSH.C) estimated using the Immulite chemiluminescent enzyme immunoassay. Sixty-eight infants had cord TSH > 25mU/L (99th centile). TSH levels (TSH.I) were measured in 45 within 48 hours of birth. TSH levels (TSH.II) were also done in 39 of them a second time after 4 days of life. TSH.I was above 20 (95th centile) in only 6 babies, and 2 of them TSH.I > TSH.C. One was subsequently diagnosed to have hypothyroidism. All others went on have normal TSH.II values. The TSH.I was done while the baby was in hospital without any inconvenience and anxiety to the parents; its discriminating ability resulted in only 6 out of the original 68 (0.15% of those screened) needing a formal recall with its attendant anxieties. We conclude that very early repeating of TSH values in those with a high cord TSH is useful in significantly decreasing formal recall rates.*

Introduction

There are reports indicating that about 5–10% of congenital hypothyroidism are not detected by the various newborn screening strategies[1]. The main reason being hormone levels that do not meet recall criteria. This source of false negatives can be controlled by adjusting recall criteria to increase sensitivity but at the cost of specificity. We have been screening newborns since 1983 using initially a primary cord serum T4 with supplemental TSH strategy, then a T4 and TSH strategy and now a primary cord serum TSH strategy with recall values of 25 mU/l (99th centile)[2,3,4] This strategy has enabled high detection rates, approximately 1 in 3000, of persistent primary hypothyroidism.

However the recall rate is high, about 1.5%. As the process of recall is associated with increased parental anxiety, significant costs and increased clinical workload and logistic demands, there is a need to reduce the recall rate.

We hypothesized that in those infants with an elevated cord TSH, a second TSH done before primary discharge (about 24–48 hours of age) will help to reduce the number who need a formal recall and thorough evaluation. This study was mounted to prove the hypothesis. As the mothers and their babies in our hospital often go home even before 24 hours of delivery, a secondary aim was to determine whether the hypothesis, if proven, was practical to implement.

Methods

The procedure involved doing a TSH level before 48 hours of age (TSH.I) and a second TSH level after 72 hours of age (TSH.II) in babies with a cord TSH level (TSH.C) that exceeded 25 mu/L. This value was our previously established cut off value for recall and corresponded to the 99th percentile value of the normal population. If more than 50% of babies had TSH.I < 20 mU/L (95th centile for age) and TSH.I < TSH.II then the hypothesis would be considered to be proved.

TSH levels were measured using the commercially available Immulite chemiluminescent enzyme immunoassay. This assay is a third generation immunometric assay which uses monoclonal TSH specific antibodies. The assay has a range of 0.002 to 75 mu/L and the coefficients of variations for the upper and lower part of the range, respectively, was, intraassay 13.8 – 4.5% and interassay 17.5 – 8 percent. The assay is completed in about 2 hours.

Results

Sixty eight babies comprising 1.5% of the 4706 live births between June 1994 and October 1995 at the National University Hospital had cord TSH values that exceeded 25 mU/L. In 45 (66%) of them it was possible for TSH.I to be determined. A TSH.II was done in 62 babies. In 39 babies both

TSH.I and TSH.II values were done, in 6 only TSH.I and in 23 only TSH.II values were done.

Among the 39 with paired TSH values, TSH.I was > 20 mU/L in 6 (15%). In 2 of the 6, TSH.I was also greater than TSH.C, one of them was subsequently diagnosed to have hypothyroidism. None of the babies with TSH.I < 20 mU/L had TSH.II > 20 mU/L.

Among the 45 with TSH.I only 6 (13%) had values greater than 20mU/l and thus needed a recall. Extrapolating this proportion to the 68 who needed a recall on the basis of an elevated cord TSH, only 9 would have needed a recall. The effective recall rate was thus 0.2% a more than 80% reduction when compared to the original 1.5% recall rate.

The TSH values and trends obtained in the 6 babies with TSH.I > 20 mU/L are distinctly different and opposite to those obtained in previously diagnosed hypothyroidism. Those in the latter being much higher and not showing any evidence of a fall in TSH values. Thus even if TSH.I is >20 mU/L, the false positive nature of a result can be confidently established by comparing the TSH.I with the TSH.C and only very rarely will a further evaluation be necessary.

Discussion

The primary task in a screening programme is the early identification of cases and institution of appropriate treatment. A secondary task which is often overlooked is for the case identification to be accomplished with the least amount of disturbance to the unaffected individual.

The cord serum based programme is associated with the highest number of false positives. This is because of the physiological TSH surge producing elevations of TSH that exceed cut off values.

Very early TSH testing (TSH.I) has been shown to be as discriminatory as late TSH testing (TSH.II). It has the advantage of being done while the child is still in hospital without much fuss and parental anxiety. The physical inconvenience associated with the bringing of a new-born baby back to the hospital is also set aside. The costs involved in bringing a baby to hospital for review can also be reduced.

The main limitation is to ensure that the baby is not sent home prior to a knowledge of the TSH.I. About 23 (34%) of those with elevated cord TSH could not have a TSH.I done because they were already home when the news of the elevated TSH.C was known. To determine the magnitude of this group we had intentionally not delayed discharge till the screening results were known. As the number involved is small we have now decided to delay discharge until the screening result is known. This usually involves only about a 1–2 hour delay and has been easily accepted by parents. This is so because the they readily appreciate the advantages of the short delay. We also do have a precedence. Our G6PD deficiency screening programme calls for discharge to be delayed until the screening result is known.

In conclusion we have shown that in newborns with elevated cord TSH levels, a TSH estimation within 48 hours of birth, readily identifies primary hypothyroidism, is useful in identifying those who do not need a recall, is practical and thus is able to reduce the recall rates to an acceptable values.

References

1. Yeo PPB, Joseph R, Chua D, et. al. Screening program for congenital hypothyroidism in Singapore. In: Naruse H, Irie N, ed. Neonatal screening, Amsterdam: Elsevier Science Publishers B.V., 1983:113–4.
2. Joseph R, Ho LY, Gomez JM, et al. Non isotopic cord serum screening for congenital hypothyroidism in Singapore — the TSH and T4 strategy. In: Wilcken B, Webster D, ed. Screening in the nineties, Australia, 8th International Neonatal Screening Symposium, 1991:69–70.
3. Joseph R, Aw TC, Tan KL. Free thyroxin as a supplement to thyrotropin in cord screening for hypothyroidism. Ann Acad Med Sin 1993;22:549–52.
4. LaFranchi S, Hanna CE, Krainz PL, et al. Screening for congenital hypothyroidism with specimen collection at two time periods: results of the Northwest regional screening programme. Ped 1985;76:734–40.

Newborn Screening for Congenital Hypothyroidism in Beijing, China

Yisheng Xi[1] *, Shunhua Li[1], Xuming Zhang[2], Lanxing Lin[2]

[1] *Newborn Screening Centre of Beijing, Beijing, China.* [2] *Beijing Institute of Child Health, Beijing, China. * Corresponding author.*

Abstract *Congenital hypothyroidism (CH) is one of the most common endocrine disorders in childhood in many populations. Thyroid defects present at birth, but clinical manifestation are not always obvious until after several months. If not treated early and appropriately, the patient will be severely mentally retarded. CH can be detected in the neonatal period by newborn screening. From July 1989 to June 1995, we found 31 cases of CH by newborn screening in Beijing, the incidence rate being 1:8385. Among the 31 patients, 10 were males and 21 females. Thyroidiea radioisotope scanning showed 8 of these 31 patients had no thyroid gland, 10 had hypoplastic thyroid gland, 3 were ectopic thyroid gland, 7 were normal and 5 had not been tested. Effects of treatment: serum T3, T4, TSH of most the 31 patients returned to normal after taking desiccated thyroid for 2–4 weeks. The children's height, listening ability and radiographs of bone wrist joints or knee joints were normal for age. Their intelligence level as tested by Gesell or DDST method was also normal. Our results further support for the need of mass neonatal screening for CH to allow early and appropriate medical intervention to the affected infants.*

Introduction

Congenital Hypothyroidism (CH) is one of the most common endocrine disorders in childhood. Thyroid defects present at birth, but clinical manifestations are not always obvious until several months. If not treated early, the patient may be severely mentally retarded. CH can be detected in the neonatal period by newborn screening. If treated early, the prognosis is greatly improved. During July 1989 to June 1995, we found 31 cases of CH by newborn screening. The methods for screening, diagnosis and treatment of these patients are reported as follows:

Methods

Working up the Beijing Newborn Screening Network   The newborn screening was started in July 1989 in Beijing under the supervision of Beijing Public Health Bureau. The headquarters of Beijing Newborn Screening Network is in the Beijing Center of Newborn Screening. The covering area of newborn screening network has been expanding. It has increased from 14.01% in 1989 to 73.67% in June 1995.

Sample collection   Prior to September 1992, umbilical cord blood samples were obtained as blood spots on filter paper by which TSH levels were determined. Later on, blood samples were collected by heel-prick 3 to 7 days after birth. The filter paper used was from DPC Company, USA, and TSH levels are determined by radioimmunoassay.

Diagnosis and Treatment   TSH level in cord blood ≥ 20 μIU/mL and in the heelblood ≥ 30 μIU/mL were defined as positive. Then for babies with positive TSH tests, serum T_3, T_4 and TSH levels were determined to confirm the diagnosis. Patients suspected with CH would be examined by thyroid radioisotope scanning to find out the basic defects. As soon as the diagnosis was made, the patients were immediately treated with desiccated thyroid. The initial dose is 10 mg per day, and adjusted according to thyroid function tests, patients' height, weight, intelligence, listening ability, comprehension and the development of bone age. These are monitored regularly.

Results

Totally 259,936 new born infants have been screened from July 1989 to June 1995. Among them, 31 CH were detected, 10 were males and 21 females, sex ratio 1:2.1. The incidence was 1:8385.

The results of thyroid radioisotope scanning   Among 31 CH patients, 8 have no thyroid gland, 8 have hypoplasis thyroid gland, 3 was ectopic thyroid gland, 7 was normal and 5 have not been tested. It seems that the majority are thyroid gland dysphasia. Some parents did not want to expose their babies to radioactive rays because they thought the children are too young. That was the reason why some patient shad not been tested.

Effect of treatment   Most of the 31 CH patients' serum T_3, T_4, TSH became normal after taking desiccated thyroid for 2–4 weeks. The

Table 1   Screening results in different years

Year	Borns	Samples	Coverage %	CH patients
1989	126840	17771	14.01	1
1990	112880	43103	38.18	6
1991	80960	34061	42.21	3
1992	82105	48009	58.47	1
1993	71644	46442	64.82	11
1994	72728	47021	64.65	4
1995	31940	23529	73.67	5
(January to June)				
Total	579099	259936		31

Table 2   The results of TSH in the first screening test

TSH	$\geq 20\ \mu IU/mL$	$\geq 50\ \mu IU/mL$	$\geq 100\ \mu IU/mL$	Total
Case	9	8	12	27
%	33.33	29.63	37.04	100

Table 3   Serum T_3, T_4 levels of CH patients identified

Case	T_3	T_4	TSH
8	DEC	DEC	INC
8	N	DEC	INC
1	DEC	N	INC
14	N	N	INC

children's height and body weight were measured regularly and were normal for age. Their intelligence level was tested by Gesell or DDST method. 20 were classified as normal and 4 were not tested because of refusal by the patients. 7 were too young to be tested but they appeared normal clinically. Radiographs of bone wrist joints or knee joints showed them to be matching with age. The listening ability was normal.

Discussion

Neonatal screening has been carried out for more than about 30 years in the world. The project was started first in Shanghai in the early 1980s and then in Beijing in the late 1980s. In different populations, the incidence of CH ranges from 1:3000 to 1:8000 live birth. Shanghai Institute of Pediatrics reported that the incidence of CH is 1:6873 in 7 cities in China during September 1991 to September 1992. The CH incidence in Beijing is 1:8385.

After early diagnosis and appropriate treatment, the physical, mental development and bone age of the 31 CH are within the normal range of the same age. Neonatal Screening not only prevents a child from development of mental retardation in a family, but it also alleviates the burden on the society and the nation.

If the level of TSH $\geq$ 50 μIU/mL in the initial screening, it should be highly alerted to the possibility of having CH, and it is necessary to contact the patient on time.

Follow-up of Infants with Congenital Hypothyroidism Detected by Neonatal Screening in Guangzhou, China

XQ Ma*, CY Song, BH Lin, XY Li

*Neonatal Screening Centre, Maternal and Neonatal Hospital, Guangzhou 510180, China. * Corresponding author.*

Abstract *We report a follow-up study of 13 patients with congenital hypothyroidism (CH) detected from 92,067 babies in a screening programme by TSH determination. The follow-up period ranged form 8 months – 6 years. 11 infants had clinical symptoms at diagnosis. In 9 infants the serum T4 concentrations were below normal (reference range 8–13 μg/dl). 9 cases had retarded bone age. 8 infants were given TC99m scan at 2 years of age: 3 were thyroid-absent, 4 had an ectopic gland and 1 had eutopic gland. The mean age at the start of treatment was 57.5 ± 24.8 days, and the starting T4 dose was 6.25 ± 0.76 mg/kg (equivalent to LT4 10.4 ± 1.27 μg/kg). In 9 infants, serum T4 at 1 year of age was 12.16 ± 2.41 μg/dl. In 7 infants, serum T4 at 2 years of age was 11.8 ± 2.85 μg/dl and their mean full-scale IQ score (FIQ), verbal and performance IQ scores (VIQ, PIQ) were 92.3 ± 11, 90.7 ± 12.8 and 93.9 ± 11.1 respectively. FIQ was significantly lower than that of standardized control (100 ± 15, P < 0.05. The low FIQ may be related to severe prenatal hypothyroidism, treatment delay and unstable bioactivity of desiccated T4. There was no close relationship between the biochemical and clinical features (P > 0.05). However, the sample number was too small for proper correlation analysis.*

Introduction

A pilot neonatal screening programme for Congenital Hypothyroidism (CH) was begun in April 1989 in Guangzhou, China. A total of 92,067 babies had been screened by December 1994. We used serum TSH measurements in our screening programme and 13 cases were found to be CH.

Subjects and Methods

13 cases of CH were detected in 92,067 babies screened for CH using either DELFIA (Pharmacia Co.) or RIA (DPC, L.A.) for TSH determination on blood-soaked filter paper and confirmed by RIA for serum T4 and TSH levels.

All the patients were followed up by an assigned pediatrician, and treated with desiccated thyroid. The initial T4 dose was 20 mg/day and dosage was increased with age in order to maintain the serum T4 concentration in the upper range of normal (10 ~ 13 µg/dl). The serum T4,TSH levels and bone age were monitored regularly and intellectual development were evaluated with the Beijing-Gesell Scale at age 0 to 3 year and with the China-Wechsler Young Children Scale of Intelligence at 4–6 year. Treatment was suspended for 1 month when the child was 2 year of age. The technatate TC99M thyroid scan was performed, and serum T4, TSH were measured in order to determine whether the patient suffered from permanent or transient hypothyroidism.

Results

13 patients (8 males and 5 females) had been followed up for 8 months to 6 years. They were all born full-term (gestational age 38 ~ 41 weeks). 7 were delivered by caesarean section (1 was born through artificial fertilization), the rest with normal delivery. The birth weight of all babies were >2500 g (2500 ~ 3800 g), 9 (69%) were over 3000 g. 11 (85%) babies had some clinical symptoms at the time of diagnosis (number of infants in parenthesis): prolonged jaundice (6), constipation (4), large tongue (4), feeding difficulty (3), cold skin (3), abdominal distension (2), umbilical hernia (1), thick dry skin (1) and hoarse cry (1). One infant, who was born by artificial fertilization, was found to have patent ductus arteriosus. The ductus was closed after treating with indomethacin.

The initial TSH values of 13 infants were all above normal, ranging from 68.7 to >330 mu/L (Table 1). In 9 infants, the serum T4 values at diagnosis were below normal (<1.0~3.5 µg/dl), and 4 were within the normal limits (reference range 8.0–13.0 µg/dl). 9 cases had retarded bone age at diagnosis; 4 were normal. Of the 8 infants who had undergone TC 99m scan, 3 showed absent thyroid; 4 had an ectopic gland; one had normal gland. The mean age of the infants when the treatment was started was 57.5 ± 24.8 days (ranging between 20 and 100 days). Only 2 cases were treated

Table 1 Clinical and biochemical features of the infants with CH

Case No	Age (Year)	Filter paper TSH mu/L	Serum T4 µg/dl	Retarded bone age	Thyroid scanning	Age started to treat (day)
1	6	114	2.8	+	Absence	23
2	5	274.8	1.9	+	Absence	20
3	3	185.6	3.5	—	Lingual	36
4	2	>253	<2.0	+	Lingual	81
5	2	113	3.0	+	Normal	40
6	2	>330	8.5	+	Absence	74
7	2	186	8.0	+	Lingual	72
8	1	240	<2.0	+	—	63
9	1	68.7	12.1	—	Lingual	66
10	1	>218	<2.0	—	—	72
11	8/12	313.7	<1.0	+	—	31
12	8/12	>314	1.9	+	—	70
13	8/12	160.5	13.0	—	—	100

* T4-RIA normal value 4.3 ~ 13 µg/dl
** TSH-RIA normal value <10 mu/L

within 1 month old. The reasons of delayed treatment were: samples were not sent in time; the tests were not done in time because of unavailability of RIA reagents, addresses were unclear or changed. The mean starting dose of desiccated thyroid was 6.25 ± 0.76 mg/kg (equivalent to LT4 10.4 ± 1.27 µg/kg). The mean serum T4 value was 9.5 ± 4.66 µg/dl (3.4~20 µg/dl) after 3~4 weeks of treatment. In 9 infants, mean serum T4 value at I year of age was 12.6 ± 2.41 µg/dl (9.9–15.4 µg/dl). In 7 infants, mean serum T4 level at 2 years of age was 11.8 ± 2.85 µg/dl (6.2–14.7 µg/dl). The mean full-scale IQ score (FIQ), verbal and performance IQ scores (VIQ, PIQ) were 92.3 ± 11, 90.7 ± 12.8 and 93.9 ± 11.1 respectively. The FIQ was significantly lower than that of standardized controls (100 ± 15, $P < 0.05$).

Discussion

In this study, 11 infants (85%) had some clinical symptoms at diagnosis, but none had been diagnosed based on these non-specific clinical symptoms without the screening results. This denotes that neonatal screening for CH is very important for early diagnosis and early treatment. Grant et al. reported a close relationship between the biochemical severity of CH and early clinical symptoms in 449 infants. But in our study, which is a relatively small-scale study, serum T4 values were not related to the clinical features, retarded bone age and thyroid agenesis ($P > 0.05$).

The mean FIQ of 7 infants at 2 years of age was significantly lower than that of the standardized control subjects. This may be due to the late treatment and unstable bioactivity of the desiccated thyroid prescribed to these infants.

Money et al.[2] followed up ten patients with CH for 16 to 26 years after an original IQ test at age 5 to 6. The mean full scale IQ was increased by 21. The data suggested that in CH intellectual growth may increase with effective hormonal replacement and education. Infants in this study should be observed more closely and intervened with early education in order to improve mental development.

Acknowledgments

We are grateful to Drs Li Hua and YL Liao for performing the development tests, statist Wang Ping for data analyses and the Department of Nuclear Medicine of Guangzhou Military General Hospital for thyroid scan. We also thank all of the colleagues participating in this screening network.

References

1. Grant DB, et al. Congenital hypothyroidism detected by neonatal screening: relationship between biochemical severity and early clinical features. Arch Dis Child 1992;67:89–90.
2. Money J, et. al. Congenital hypothyroidism and IQ increase: A quarter century follow-up. J Pediatr 1978;93:432–34.

Neonatal Screening Programme for Congenital Hypothyroidism in Hong Kong

KK Lo, Stephen TS Lam*

*Neonatal Screening Unit, Clinical Genetic Service, Department of Health, Cheung Sha Wan Jockey Club Clinic, Shamshuipo, Hong Kong.   * Corresponding author.*

Abstract   Studies in the early seventies had proved that congenital hypothyroidism (CH) could be detected in early neonatal period by screening programme and early replacement treatment with thyroxine was possible. The neonatal screening programme for CH was started in Hong Kong in March 1984 by measurement of cord blood TSH. Babies with elevated TSH were evaluated again at Day 5. Those with persistent elevated TSH were investigated for CH by full physical investigation, X-ray for bone maturation, anti-thyroid antibody and technetium thyroid scan. Between 26 March 1984 and 30 June 1995, 451,391 new-borns (233,612 male and 217,779 female) were screened for CH. The coverage was 100% for the target population. 145 babies (51 male and 94 female, ratio being 1 to 1.84) were diagnosed to have CH, the incidence was thus 1 in 3,113 live-births. Technetium thyroid scan were performed in 139 cases, 6.5% (9 cases) had thyroid agenesis, 49.6% (69 cases) had ectopic thyroid and the remaining 43.9% (61 cases) had normal thyroid scan. 99 cases were reassessed at the age of 3 years. 23 cases were proven to be having transient hypothyroidism and they all had normal thyroid scan. The mean age of starting thyroxine replacement therapy was 21 days (range 4 to 195 days). We conclude that neonatal screening programme for CH plays a significant role in the prevention of mental retardation.

Introduction

Congenital hypothyroidism is a common cause of mental retardation and short stature affecting about 1 in 4000 newborns in most populations. Early treatment with thyroxine replacement can effectively prevent mental and physical retardations. However, diagnosis in the neonatal period on clinical grounds is difficult because there are little signs and symptoms. With the development of highly sensitive radioimmunoassay for determination of thyroxine (T4) and thyroid stimulating hormone (TSH), it was possible to detect congenital hypothyroidism by neonatal screening. Experiences of neonatal screening for congenital hypothyroidism in Quebec, Canada[1] and Pittsburgh, USA[2] in early seventies confirmed the value of screening programme in early detection and replacement therapy. The high incidence of congenital hypothyroidism justified this programme on a cost effectiveness basis.

Method

The neonatal screening programme for congenital hypothyroidism was started in Hong Kong in March 1984. The programme covered most of the babies born in the public institutions. By 1995, it covered 10 hospitals administered under the Hospital Authority of Hong Kong and 6 government maternity homes, which represent the majority of all newborns delivered in the public sector.

2.5 ml cord blood was taken at birth at the placental side in a plain bottle. The sample was delivered to the neonatal screening laboratory and TSH assayed by a immunoradiometric technique. The use of cord blood ensured high acceptance of the test by parents. However, the greater variations in TSH values make it necessary to allow a lower cut off level and hence a higher recall rate. Newborns with cord blood TSH level higher than the 5th percentile were assayed for T4 level and the babies were recalled for further evaluation at day 5 after birth. At recall visit, a medical history was taken with particular attention to family history of thyroid diseases and maternal administration of antithyroid drugs. The babies were examined for signs and symptoms of congenital hypothyroidism (Table 1) and venous blood taken for TSH and T4 assay. Those with persistent high TSH and low T4 levels were further investigated for congenital hypothyroidism which included X-ray for bone maturation, anti-thyroid antibody and radioactive technetium thyroid scan. Confirmed cases of congenital hypothyroidism were given replacement therapy with L-thyroxine after thyroid scan and were referred back to paediatricians for follow up and continued treatment.

Patients were reassessed at the age of three years to determine the persistence of hypothyroidism. Thyroid hormone replacement was temporarily suspended, TSH and T4 assays were performed 4 weeks after T4 was taken off. Radioactive thyroid scan were performed in selected cases.

Table 1 Age of starting thyroxine replacement therapy for patient with congenital hypothyroidism

Age at which treatment begin (weeks)	Number of Patients	Cumulative Number
1	17	17 (12%)
2	63	80 (55%)
3	23	103 (71%)
4	17	120 (83%)
5	10	130 (90%)
6	4	134 (92%)
>6	11	145 (100%)

Children with normal thyroid function were labelled as transient congenital hypothyroidism and treatment discontinued.

Results

During the twelve years period from 26 March 1984 to 30 June 1995, 451,391 newborns (233,612 males and 217,779 females) were screened for congenital hypothyroidism, which represented almost 100% of all the newborns in this population. 145 cases of congenital hypothyroidism were detected, giving an incidence rate of 1 in 3,113 live-births. There were 51 males and 94 females, male to female ratio being 1 to 1.84.

Technetium thyroid scan were performed in 139 cases. 49.6% (69 cases) had ectopic thyroid, 6.5% (9 cases) had thyroid agenesis and 43.9% (61 cases) had normal thyroid scan. The mean age of starting thyroxine replacement was 21 days, ranging from 4 to 195 days (Table 1). The patient with treatment started at 195 days after birth had good compensated hypothyroidism until 7 months of age. Subsequent follow up at three years revealed him to be having transient hypothyroidism and treatment was stopped.

104 babies was born between the period 26 March 1984 to 30 June 1992. Reassessment at age of three years was performed for 99 cases. 23 cases had normal thyroid function and thus transient congenital hypothyroidism. All patients with transient congenital hypothyroidism had normal thyroid scan.

Discussion

Our study showed that the incidence of congenital hypothyroidism is

1:3,113 which is similar to results obtained in other countries. The female dominance is also observed as in other studies, the cause of which is unknown.

Most babies delivered in Hong Kong were discharged home very early and may not return to maternal and child health centre before the first month. The use of cord blood assay ensured a high acceptance rate and the procedure itself is non-invasive. The disadvantages of cord blood assay were a higher recall rate and screening for many inborn errors of metabolism might not be conveniently incorporated into the programme. The implementation of neonatal screening allowed early detection and early therapy for congenital hypothyroidism. In our study, more than 90% of all cases had diagnosis and treatment within the first six week after birth. For the remaining cases, all had well compensated hypothyroidism during the neonatal period and subsequent follow up showed that they suffered from transient hypothyroidism.

Transient hypothyroidism occurred in 23 case out of 104 patients, represent 22% of all cases of congenital hypothyroidism. The figure was high when compared with other studies. This may be attributed to the low cut off point for TSH level in our study. We detected very mild compensated hypothyroidism which may be missed if a higher TSH cut off level had been used.

A previous study[3] showed that children with congenital hypothyroidism had psychomotor developmental delay despite treatment, especially those with low initial T4 level, delayed bone maturation at diagnosis and thyroid agenesis. In our study, mental assessment at age 3 and 5 years of age were performed in selected cases. Preliminary result did not show any significant mental deficit (data not showed).

In summary, our experience in neonatal screening for congenital hypothyroidism showed that the programme contributes towards prevention of mental and physical handicap.

References

1. Dussault JH, Coulombe P, Laberge C, et el. Preliminary report on a mass screening program for neonatal hypothyroidism. J Pediatr 1975;86:670–4.
2. Klein AH, Augustin AV, Folwy TP Jr. Successful screening for congenital hypothyroidism. Lancet 1974;2:77–9.
3. Rovet J, Ehrich R, Sorbara D. Intellectual outcome in children with fetal hypothyroidism. J Pediatr 1987;110:700–4.

Congenital Hypothyroidism Presenting with Mildly Elevated Thyrotropin in the Cord Blood

Connie FT Sham, Stephen TS Lam*

*Clinical Genetic Service, Department of Health, Cheung Sha Wan Jockey Club Clinic, Shamshuipo, Kowloon, Hong Kong.   * Corresponding author.*

Abstract   *Hong Kong is one of the few places in the world where cord blood serum thyrotropin level is used for screening of congenital hypothyroidism. From 1984 to 1991, 95 babies were confirmed to have congenital hypothyroidism. With a low cutoff level of 14 to 17 mIU/L, there was a high false positive rate and a high recall rate of 6%. Out of the 95 babies, 9 cases were identified in which the cord blood thyrotropin level were 20 mIU/L, and their congenital hypothyroidism were subsequently proved to be transient and of a mild degree. An attempt to increase the cord serum thyrotropin cutoff so as to decrease the false positive rate would have lead to these 9 cases being missed. Whether the low cutoff level is justified is discussed.*

Introduction

The neonatal screening programme for congenital hypothyroidism (CHT) was started in 1984 by the Hong Kong Government. Cord blood was collected for screening for 2 reasons. The first is that there is concomitant screening for glucose-6-phosphate dehydrogenase and the availability of early results would be beneficial. The second reason was that a considerable proportion of newborn babies were discharged from the hospitals early, so that the collection of postnatal blood samples for screening would be difficult. The cord blood samples were assayed for serum thyrotropin(TSH) level using the immunoradiometric method. Babies with serum TSH above the cutoff value in the cord blood were recalled for clinical assessment and repeat blood testing on day 5 of age and were managed accordingly.

From 1984 to 1991, the TSH cutoff was set at 14 to 17 mIU/L. 303,057 babies were screened and 95 babies were confirmed to have congenital hypothyroidism with a recall rate of 6% and an incidence of congenital hypothyroidism of 1 in 3190. In an attempt to decrease the recall rate, the 95 confirmed cases of CHT were studied in detail, and 9 babies presenting with only mildly elevated TSH in the cord blood were identified.

Materials and Method

95 babies with CHT were born in different hospitals from 1984 to 1991. The diagnosis of CHT was made after an initial workup including thyroid function test, x-rays for bone age and technetium thyroid scan. The thyrotropin(TRH) stimulating test and ultrasound scan of the thyroid gland were performed on selected cases. The babies were referred back to the paediatricians of the hospitals in which they were born for subsequent management and follow-up. All babies with an anatomically normal thyroid gland on initial workup were assessed at the age of 3 years or earlier for the need of lifelong thyroxine treatment. During the assessment, thyroid function test and technetium thyroid scan were performed with thyroxine replacement stopped. Babies with TSH and T4 level remaining within normal limits after thyroxine replacement were stopped were diagnosed as transient hypothyroidism.

Data were retrieved from the hospital files of these 95 babies retrospectively.

Results

Of the 95 babies with CHT, 60% were found to have thyroid agenesis or an ectopic thyroid gland, 24% were found to suffer from transient hypothyroidism with thyroxine replacement stopped at or before 3 years of age, the remaining 16% were found to have a normal thyroid gland on scan but treatment could not be stopped.

9 babies were found to have serum TSH level of 20 mIU/L in the cord blood while the rest had serum TSH level of >30 mIU/L in the cord blood. The clinical data of the 9 cases with mildly elevated TSH in the cord blood were summarized in Table 1. The serum TSH level before thyroxine replacement was started were plotted in the graph in Figure 1.

Discussion

Cord blood TSH level has been known to have a wider variation in

Table 1 9 cases of CHT presenting with mildly elevated TSH level in the cord blood

Case No.	1	2	3	4	5	6	7	8	9
Sex	M	F	F	F	M	F	F	M	F
Birth weight (kg)	2.6	2.5	2.1	3.1	3.3	3.1	3	3.4	3.9
Gestation	36 weeks	term	36 weeks	term	term	term	term	term	term
*TSH/T4 results									
• cord blood	• 18/91	• 17/86	• 17/124	• 20/139	• 16/152	• 15/101	• 14/84	• 20/107	• 19/118
• 1st week	• 117/40	• 55/96	• 21/152	• 66/96	• —	• 52/82	• 26/144	• 43/111	• 63/60
• 2nd week	• 9/102	• —	• —	• —	• 48/137	• 151/47	• 40/91	• 30/123	• 156/38
• just before T4 started	• 107/51 (6th week)	• 109/67 (4th week)	• 174/49 (4th week)	• 260/38 (4th week)	• 160/65 (11th week)		• 80/74 (5th week)	• 107/79 (7th week)	• —
Bone age at birth	36 weeks	term	36 weeks	38 weeks	2.5 months (taken at 10 weeks of age)	term	38–40 weeks	term	term
Thyroid scan	normal	normal	normal	normal	normal	normal	normal	normal	normal
Age when thyroxine was started	6 week	5 week	5 week	4 week	11 week	3 week	5 week	8 week	4 week
Age when thyroxine was stopped	3 year	4 year	3 year	3 year	2.5 year	3 year	3 year	2 year	1.5 year
Highest dose of thyroxine given	?	25 µg QD	25 µg QD	25 µg QD	?	?	25 µgQD	25 µg alternate day	25 µg QD
Physical development	normal	normal	normal	normal	normal	normal	normal	normal	normal
Mental development	normal	normal	normal	normal	normal	normal	normal	normal	normal

• TSH in mIU/L, T4 in nmol/L

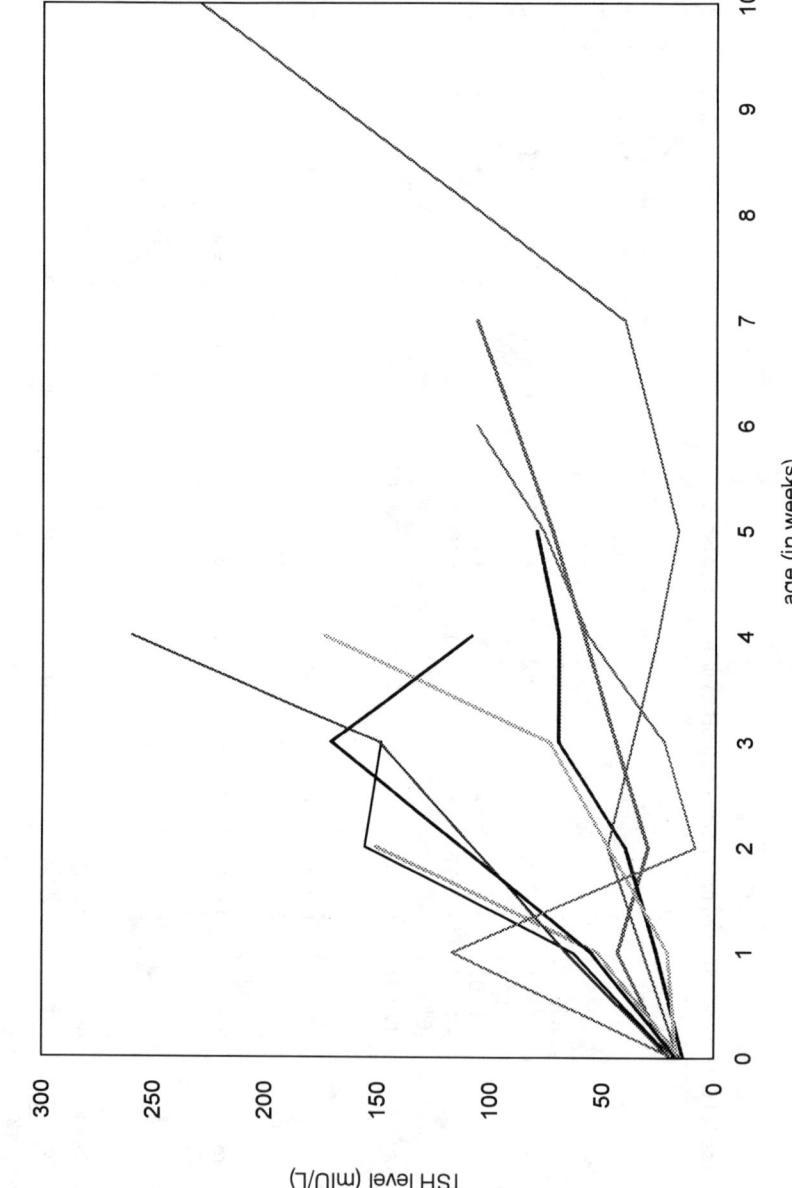

Figure 1 9 Cases of CHT presenting with mildly elevated cord blood TSH — serum TSH before thyroxine replacement was started.

normal range when compared to postnatal samples. It has been reported to be influenced by factor such as mode of delivery[1], and has been suggested to be related to the stress of difficult or complicated delivery in the healthy newborns[2].

For the screening programme in Hong Kong from 1984 to 1991, there was a 6% recall rate which meant that around 18,000 babies were recalled. For every confirmed case of CHT, 190 babies were recalled for assessment on day 5 of age. While it had been demonstrated that the parents of neonates with false positive results harboured a significantly higher anxiety level[3], the workload on the screening staff was also tremendous. It was in an attempt to lower the recall rate when these 9 cases of CHT presenting with mildly raised TSH level in the cord blood were identified. They were found to share similar characteristics, i.e. (i) appropriate bone age at birth, (ii) normal thyroid anatomy on thyroid scan, (iii) thyroxine replacement could be stopped at or before 3 years of age, (iv) of the 6 cases in which the dosage of thyroxine replacement was known, it was never higher than 25 μg per day, (v) normal physical and mental development. These all indicated that these 9 cases suffered from CHT which was transient and of a mild degree.

Albeit the mild and transient nature of the CHT that these 9 babies were suffering, it would still be difficult to predict the outcome of the physical and mental developments if they were not treated at all, or if treatment was delayed until clinical signs and symptoms of CHT appeared. Detection of these CHT children would have been missed if a higher cutoff level of cord blood TSH had been used. On the other hand, would an alternative method be useful to identify them? It has been advocated that the routine collection of a second blood sample at 4 to 6 weeks of age for screening of CHT could detect the group of infants with delayed rise in TSH postulated to be due to animmature pituitary-thyroid negative feedback relationship. It was reported that this second screening could lead to a detection rate of 1:25,505[4]. While it may not be justified or cost-effective to set up a second screening programme when the first is effective enough provided that the TSH cutoff is set sufficiently low. The collection of blood sample from infants at 4 to 6 weeks of age would also be difficult. From the experience of other CHT screening programme, a better alternative is to use postnatal sample, preferably that of day 5, for screening of CHT.

Conclusions

We conclude that for the present situation in Hong Kong, it is justified to keep the cord blood TSH cutoff at the present low level in order to detect this special group of infants with CHT presenting with mild elevated cord blood TSH. Efforts to further characterize this group of infants and investigate into the possibility of using day 5 blood sample for screening should be continued.

References

1. Lao TT, Panesar NS. Neonatal thyrotropin and mode of delivery. Brit J Obstet Gynaeco 1989;96:1224–7.
2. Lao TT, Li CY, Panesar NS. Transient neonatal hyperthyrotropinaemia. Early Hum Devel 1992;28:19–25.
3. Tsui MKM, Lee JWK, Lam STS. Parental reaction of false positive screening test for congenital hypothyroidism. HK J Paediatr 1994;11:128–32.
4. LaFranchi SH, Hanna CE, Krainz PL, et al. Screening for congenital hypothyroidism with specimen collection at two time periods: results of the Northwest Regional Screening Program. Paediatr 1985;76:734–40.

Two Year Follow-up Study of Parental Reaction to False Positive Screening Test for Congenital Hypothyroidism

Kitty CK Li[1], Mike KM Tsui[1], John WK Lee[2], Stephen TS Lam[1] *

[1] Clinical Genetic Service, Department of Health, Cheung Sha Wan Jockey Club Clinic, Shamshuipo, Hong Kong. [2] Department of Psychiatry, Kwai Chung Hospital, Lai Chi Kwok, Hong Kong. * Corresponding author.

Abstract In 1993, we did a study on the parental reaction to false-positive screening test for congenital hypothyroidism. The result has shown that parents of neonates with suspected congenital hypothyroidism had a higher anxiety level than the control group. It was probably the immediate psychological reaction towards the iatrogenic alarm. These parents were investigated 2 years later for any lasting psychological sequelae incurred. This 2 year follow-up study demonstrated that lasting anxiety was unlikely to persist in non-specific situations, but it would affect the parental relationship, mental status and parent-child relationship in various specific hypothetical situations on a long-term basis.

Introduction

Neonatal screening of congenital hypothyroidism has proved to be effective in the prevention of mental retardation arising from untreated hypothyroidism by early diagnosis and appropriate treatment. However screening is not without cost. It can have psychological impact on the parents induced by an iatrogenic alarm[1]. In the study we carried out in 1993 on the parental reaction to false-positive screening test for congenital hypothyroidism, we have demonstrated that the parents of neonates with suspected congenital hypothyroidism harboured a significantly higher anxiety level than the control group[2]. The present study is a 2-year follow-up study of any lasting psychological sequelae incurred on these parents.

Methodology

Subjects   In the 1993 study, parents of 29 families were shown to have a high anxiety level. These parents were contacted again for the present study. Out of these 29 families, only 12 families took part in this 2-year follow-up study. The reasons for the drop-out were as follows: 1 baby died and the parents did not want to be reminded of the tragedy; 7 families had moved away and could not be contacted; 4 mothers and babies were in China; and parents of 5 families refused to attend saying that they were busy at work and could not get a day off.

Procedure   Parents were contacted by phone and invited to attend an interview at the Genetics Clinic. During interview, they were assessed by the following instruments.

A. Quantitative

Parental psychological reaction were assessed by the Hamilton Rating Scale for anxiety by one of the authors (Tsui)[3]. This scale had been used in the last study. The same scale was used in this study. It is an observer-rated semiquantitative scale constructed with 14 items to assess the severity of anxiety signs and symptoms in the past 2 weeks. Majority are symptoms based on patients' complaints. It gives information on general anxiety level. Scores of Hamilton Rating Scales for anxiety were recorded and compared with the result in 1993 study.

B. Qualitative

A questionnaire was designed for the parents to complete. It was administered by another author (Li). It consisted of 26 hypothetical questions to assess the lasting effects of false alarm on the parents' mental status, parental relationship and the parent-child relationship. It could give rise to more information about the parental response in addition to that derived from quantitative result. Answers of individual questions were analyzed and interpretations were formulated according to the response arisen during those specific hypothetical situations.

Results

A. Quantitative:

For the general anxiety level, all parents scored zero on the Hamilton

Rating Scale for anxiety. In comparison with the scores recorded in the 1993 study, statistically significant differences could be detected. ($P \ll 0.001$).

Comparison of parental anxiety level in the 1993 Study and present study based on Hamilton Rating Scales for Anxiety

Family	1993 Study		Present Study	
	Mother	Father	Mother	Father
S392	10	10	0	0
S397	12	5	0	—
S401	8	7	0	0
S403	5	0	0	—
S405	3	—	0	0
S409	9	—	0	—
S411	16	5	0	—
S416	15	16	0	0
S418	4	4	0	—
S424	2	2	0	—
S425	3	3	0	0
S433	4	4	0	—

B. Qualitative:

Some families showed presence of lasting psychological sequelae upon some hypothetical specific situations set in the questionnaire. The questionnaire was divided into 3 parts : parents' mental status, parental relationship and parent-child relationship.

1. Parents' mental status:

— **Fears of unknown (5 families — 41.6%)**
Some parents still had fears without being aware of the origin but these might not be clinically significant or related to false alarm.

— **Emotional flashback experience (3 families — 25%)**
False alarm still recurred in their mind spontaneously upon hearing telephone rings (the news of raised TSH were made known to them telephone) or seeing newborn babies .These experiences would prevent parents from working through the psychological pain.

— **Guilty feelings (3 families — 25%)**
Some mothers sometimes suspected themselves having done

something during the antenatal periods. They also condemned themselves for not the baby well if he (she) was ill .This might predispose to depressed mood of mothers, if persistent and left unattended.

— **Inability to talk about the false alarm (6 families — 50%)**
One father and five mothers would not reveal this experience to friends and they didn't want others to know. This was due to guilt feelings on the parents and their inability to integrate the experience.

— **Affecting future family planning (4 families — 33.3%)**
Some parents had anticipatory anxiety of future babies and one couple even decided not to have further pregnancies. The false alarm had altered parents' decision-making on family planning and laid down some permanent fear in their mind.

2.   Parental relationship

Anger was displaced towards the mothers: 2 husbands put the blame on their spouses when the baby was ill and related the false alarm to mothers' fault. These behaviour again put the mothers to lots of psychological distress.

3.   Parent-child relationship

Overprotection of the babies or dislike of the babies: parents of 6 families showed overconcern and tended to overprotect these babies. Another 2 couples thought that the baby was a bit troublesome. These behaviour reflected the impact of the false alarm on the rearing pattern of babies by parents. This in turn might impair the psychological development of babies e.g. immature and dependent children or rebellious children.

Discussion

This study included only parents who have taken part in the 1993 study and who have a higher anxiety level. The results demonstrate that the high anxiety level in parents incurred immediately by iatrogenic alarm is unlikely to persist in the long run. However it would affect the parental relationship, parents' mental status and parent-child relationship in various specific hypothetical situations on a long term basis.

Health counselling had been given to all involved couples, including those with false positive results before the test was repeated and that they were informed that the repeated results were normal later. It is remarkable that after 2 years, 3 families still had guilty feelings of blaming themselves for anything happening to the baby. And that half of the 12 families would never touch this subject again. They never revealed this experience to others and half of them had overprotected their babies amongst other siblings. It is doubtful that how much information from the health counselling they had understood. These parents might have coped better had they been more prepared in the ante-natal period. The study is of a small sample size. It would be better to have a wider coverage of hypothetical questions to collect more detailed information. However, these results are in line with other overseas long-term follow-up studies, so the psychological reactions of the participants in the screening programme should be seriously considered before implementation.

References

1. Marteau TM, Psychological cost of screening. Brit Med J 1989;299:527.
2. Tsui MKM, Lee JWK, Lam STS. Parental reaction of false positive screening test for congenital hypothyroidism. HK J Paed 1994;11:128–32.
3. Hamilton M. The assessment of anxiety state by rating. B J Psych 1959;32:50.
4. Bodegard G Fryo K, Larrson A. Psychological reaction in 102 families with a newborn who has a falsely positive screening test for congenital hypothyroidism. Acta Paediatr Scand 1982 Suppl;304:1–21.
5. Fyro K, Bodegard G. Four year follow-up of psychological reaction to false positive screening tests for congenital hypothyroidism. Acta Paediatr Scand 1987;76:107–14.

New Technologies

Simultaneous Analysis of Amino Acids and Acylcarnitines by Electrospray Ionization and Tandem Mass Spectrometry

Fumio Inoue*, Naoki Kodo, Naoto Terada, Masakazu Okochi , Akihiko Kinugasa, Tadashi Sawada

*Department of Pediatrics, Kyoto Prefectural University of Medicine, 465 Kajiicho, Kawaramachi-Hirokoji, Kamikyo-ku, Kyoto 602, Japan. * Corresponding author.*

Abstract *Many inherited metabolic diseases can be detected by plasma amino acid and acylcarnitine analysis in the neonatal period. We developed a method for simultaneous analysis of amino acids and acylcarnitines by electrospray ionization tandem mass spectrometry (ESI/MS/MS). Two 6 mm discs punched from a Guthrie card were incubated in methanol solution containing stable isotope labelled internal standards. An aliquot of the methanol solution was then evaporated. After butylation, amino acids and acylcarnitines were extracted by ion paired extraction. Dried extract was reconstituted by 50% acetonitrile. An aliquot was analyzed by a triple quadrupole mass spectrometer (QUATTRO, VG Biotech) equipped with an electrospray ionization source. The mobile phase was 50% acetonitrile. Acylcarnitines were analyzed by parent ion scan of m/z 85 and amino acids by neutral loss scan of m/z 102 and m/z 119. Semi-quantitative determination was conducted and resulted in good reproducibility and recovery both in amino acids and acylcarnitines. This method should be considered as one of the tools for neonatal mass screening programme.*

Introduction

For neonatal mass screening, accurate and informative methods of analysis are required. Here we describe a new method for simultaneous, confirmative and quantitative analysis of amino acids and acylcarnitines in blood spots using electrospray ionization tandem mass spectrometry (ESI-MS/MS). This method was found to be robust and reliable.

Methods

Sample preparation   Two 6 mm discs punched from the blood spots on Guthrie cards were soaked in methanol solution containing internal standards (deutrium labeled amino acids and acylcarnitines). The methanol solution was transferred to a small vial and evaporated to dryness under a nitrogen stream. To the residue 100 µl of butanol/HCl was added, and heated at 65°C for 15 min. After cooling to room temperature, 200 µl of propanol, 100 µl of water and 5 µl of 30%KI were added. Butylated amino acids and acylcarnitines were extracted two times by 200 µl of chloroform. The chloroform layer was dried, and residue was reconstituted by 50% acetonitril containing 0.2% formic acid, and an aliquot (usually 5 µl) was used for analysis by tandem MS.

Mass spectrometry   A triple quadrupole mass spectrometer (QUATTRO, VG Biotech) equipped with a electrospray ionization source was employed using 50% acetonitril in water as mobile phase. Acylcarnitines were analyzed by parent ion scan of m/z85 and amino acids analyzed by neutral loss scan of m/z102 and m/z119. Ion mass data were obtained in continuum mode, and 20 spectra were averaged, smoothed and background subtracted. Peak height was used for quantification.

Results

Acylcarnitines   Butyrated acylcarnitines were well detected by tandem mass spectrometry using the mode of parent ion scan of m/z 85. Acetylcarnitine was the main component of acylcarnitines in normal human subjects. Calibration curves for acetylcarnitine and isovalerylcarnitine had good linearity. Propionylcarnitine was prominent in methylmalonic acidemia, and isovalerylcarnitine was increased in glutaric aciduria type II. Five consecutive injections at 3 minutes intervals showed no interference between each injection.

Amino acids   Butyrated amino acids were detected by MS/MS utilizing the mode of neutral loss scan of m/z102. Glycine, alanine, leucine, isoleucine, phenylalanine and tyrosine were measured by stable isotope dilution analysis and resulted in good linearity. Coefficient of variation ranged from 10 to 20%, that was not enough for accurate quantification. Recovery of known amount of compounds added to whole blood subsequently spotted to filter cards was around 90%. The peak of phenylalanine was prominent in phenylketonuria. Phenylalanine levels obtained by this method had a good agreement with those by HPLC (r = 0.786).

Discussion

The incidences of most inherited metabolic diseases are low. Therefore neonatal mass screening programme for metabolic diseases in Japan has low cost performance. Simultaneous detection of many kinds of inherited metabolic diseases will improve cost performance. Reliable methods of analysis will also improve test performance for avoiding false positive or negative results. The incidences of various organic acidemia have been increasing since gas chromatography mass fragementography (GCMS) has been introduced for the analysis of urinary organic acids. Several organic acidemias have higher incidences than amino acid disorders, and some of them can be diagnosed by acylcarnitine analysis, including propionic acidemia, methylmalonic acidemia and short-chain and long-chain acyl-CoA dehydrogenase deficiencies. Simultaneous analysis of amino acids and acylcarnitines by ESI-MS/MS require shorter analytical time and yield more information than conventional GCMS analysis. However quantitative data showed large coefficient of variation showing not too satisfactory precision. Since automation of several analytical steps is possible, the imprecision should be much improved after further optimization. This method may be a excellent candidate for neonatal mass screening in future.

Conclusion

Simultaneous analysis of amino acids and acylcarnitines by ESI-MS/MS was performed in blood spot on Guthrie cards obtained by neonatal mass screening. Profiling of amino acids and acylcarnitines provided gave important information for diagnosis. Quantitative analysis had some difficulty for accurate measurement both in amino acids and acylcarnitines, and more improvement on the analytical technique should be needed for quantification. Automation and optimization of several steps in the analytical procedure will enable this method to be a candidate for future neonatal mass screening programmes.

References

1. Millington DS, Kodo N, Norwood DL, Roe CR. Tandem mass spectrometry: a new method for acylcarnitine profiling with potential for neonatal screening for inborn errors of metabolism. J Inher Metab Dis 1990;13:321–4.
2. Chase DH, Millington DS, Terada N, Kahler SG, Roe CR, Hoffman LF. Rapid diagnosis of phenylketonuria by quantitative analysis of phenylalanine and tyrosine in neonatal blood spots by tandem mass spectrometry. Clin Chem 1993;38:1–6.
3. Rashed MS, Ozand PT, Bucknall MP, Little D. Diagnosis of inborn errors of metabolism from blood spots by acylcarnitines amino acids profiling using automated electrospray tandem mass spectrometry. Pediatr Res 1995;38:324–31.

Advanced Microfluorometry for Newborn Metabolic Screening

Akihiro Yamaguchi[1]*, Masaru Fukushi[1], Yasumasa Sato[1], Yuko Kikuchi[1], Harumi Ohtake[2], Akie Fujimoto[2], Tosiaki Oura[2] and Yutaka Hase[3]

[1] *Sapporo City Institute of Public Health, Sapporo, Japan.* [2] *Osaka City Environment and Public Health Association, Osaka, Japan.* [3] *Osaka City Turumi Health Center, Osaka, Japan.* *Corresponding author*

Abstract *We report the use of microfluorometry (MFL) for newborn screening of phenylketonuria (PKU), maple syrup urine disease (MSUD), homocystinuria (HCU) and galactosemia (GE) as an alternative method for bioassay which may give ambiguous results. MFL is developed as a fully quantitative method to obtain simple and objective results by chemical or enzymatic fluorogenic reactions in microplates. The assay conditions have been optimized to detect metabolites in dried blood spots: phenylalanine for PKU, branched-chain amino acids (BRAA) for MSUD, methionine (MET) and total homocysteine (HSH) for HCU, galactose (GAL) and gal-1-phosphate for GE. For GAL and BCAA assays a coupled enzymatic reaction with resazurin/ diaphorase was used and gave resorfine fluorescence with high sensitivity and specificity. For HCU screening, a method was developed using methionine γ-lyase, which measured the sum of MET and HSH and is more reliable to detect newborn HCU patients. Semi-automation was achieved by using a punch indexer model VII Jr. (Fundamentals), an auto-reagent delivery system MegaFlex (Tecan) and a fluorometric microplate reader Fluoroskan II (Labsystems). The proposed MFL system is reliable and easy for newborn metabolic screening and provide sufficient capacity for multiple assays of large number of samples.*

Introduction

Bacterial inhibition assays: Guthrie[1] and Paigen phage[2] methods have been widely used since the 1960s for the newborn screening for inborn errors of metabolism including phenylketonuria (PKU), maple syrup urine disease (MSUD), homocystinuria (HCU) and galactosemia (GE). These bioassays have sufficient capability and sensitivity. They do not need heavy and expensive instrumentation. The positive bacterial growth is suitable for identification by visual inspection. However, it is difficult to quantify and there is always the need for objective evaluation. To overcome these disadvantages other techniques providing quantitative results have been used and established on autoanalyzers[3], high performance liquid chromatography (HPLC)[4] or tandem mass spectrometry (MS-MS)[5]. These sophisticated methods, however, can only handle a limited number of samples. In contrast, microfluorometry (MFL) consists of fluorogenic reactions and measurements in the same microplate wells has sufficient sample capacity for the multiple screening with fully objective results[6,7,8]. It is also a fast method with capability of automation. We describe here advanced MFL which has been improved from the previous systems.

Methods

The assay conditions are summarized in Table 1. Indicative metabolites in dried blood spots are: Phe for PKU, Met plus total homocysteine (HSH) for HCU, branched-chain amino acids (BCA) for MSUD, and Gal plus Gal-1-P for GE. Ninhydrin-peptide method is most reliably used for Phe as in previous MFL. In Gal and BCA assays, UV fluorescence of NADH; a product of each dehydrogenase reaction was directly measured in previous MFL, now it is derived to resorfine fluorescence adopting a coupled enzymatic reaction with resazurin/diaphorase[9]. HSH alone was measured previously screening by a chemical method. Here, a new enzymatic

Table 1 Summary of Advanced MFL

Disease	Method	Measured	Cut-off (mg/dl)
Phenylketonuria	Ninhydrin Peptide	Phe	2.5
Homocystinuria	Met-lyase/OPA-2ME	HSH, Met	2.5
Maple syrup urine disease	LeuDH/Resourfine	Leu, Ile, Val	8.5
Galactosemia	GalDH/Resourufine	Gal, Gal-1-P	6.0

Improvement of previous Microfluorometry
1. Nonspecific fluorescence is eliminated in Gal and BCA assays by adopting resorfine system in combination with NADH system.
2. Reliable enzymatic assay for sum of Met and HSH is newly developed instead of a chemical method for HSH alone.
3. Automated reagent delivery system and fluorometric microplate reader of the rigid type are introduced.

assay10 for sum of Met and HSH was developed by the use of methionine g-lyase. Ammonium; a stoichiometric product of Met or HSH by the enzymatic reaction was determined subsequently by a specific reaction with o-phthalaldehyde and 2-mercaptoethanol (OPA/2ME) at neutral pH.

Practical semi-automation is achieved by introducing instruments designated for microplate use such as punch indexer model VII Jr. (Fundamentals), an auto-reagent delivery system MegaFlex (Tecan) and fluorometric microplate reader Fluoroskan II (Labsystems). The auto-reagent delivery system is adopted newly and the microplate reader for a rigid microplate are replaced the previous one limited for a stripped well microplate. These 4 assays of MFL for several hundreds of samples could be completed within a half day providing fully calculated results by a single technician.

Results and Discussion

The calibration curves and calculated outputs of newborn samples in typical routine MFL were shown in Figure 1, 2. Calibration curves were all linear and the newborn results were distributed uniformly showing no systematic deviations within a plate (96 wells) or between plates. The last 3 samples in each assay were controls spiked with the indicative metabolite at 3 concentration levels. All newborn samples in these assays were lower than the cut-off values except for some samples in Gal assay. Positive samples in MFL are submitted to confirmatory tests before request the second specimen in our screening system such as the fractional determination of Gal and Gal-l-P with transferase and epimerase enzyme activities tests for Gal or HPLC determination of aminoacids for others. Under the cut-off values shown in Table 1 the percentage of the sample submitted to the confirmatory tests are less than 5% for Gal and less than 1% in each of others.

Non specific fluorescence caused by air or dust contaminants were used to be encountered in NADH fluorescence measurements of Gal and BCA assays especially when a reflective type reader for a rigid microplate was used. This phenomenon could be completely eliminated by adopting resorfine fluorometry which gives longer emission wavelength than NADH. This modification improves specificity in Gal and BCA assays and uses the rigid type microplate reader which is much easier to handle than the stripped type microplate reader used before.

Some false negative cases were reported in newborn screening for

Figure 1 Calibration Curves in MFL

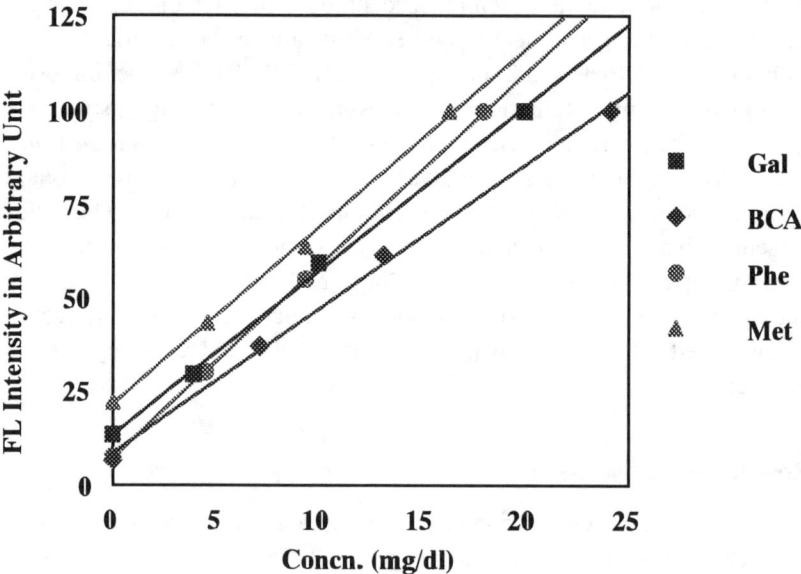

Figure 2 Typical Outputs of MFL

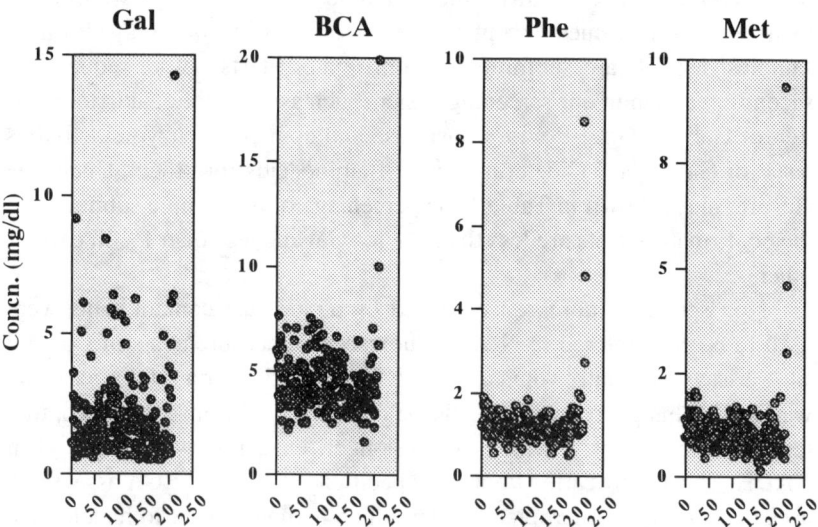

HCU by measuring Met using the Guthrie method. From the metabolic pathways the primarily accumulated metabolites in HCU should be HSH. Increase Met is secondary. We had previously designed a new assay to measure HSH by a chemical method in MFL. However, the exact measurements of HSH in dried blood spots was difficult because of the poor recovery of HSH (around 50%) in addition to its low physiological concentrations. An advanced MFL using an enzymatic assay for total Met and HSH was developed and was retrospectively proved to be able to detect 3 newborn patients with HCU whose Met levels were 2 to 8 mg/dl-blood by the Guthrie method at age 5 or 6 days after birth. The new method is expected to be more sensitive than the previous methods measuring Met or HSH alone.

Semi-automated system of MFL consists of specified instruments; the punch indexer, auto-reagent delivery system and the rigid type-microplate reader enables to save man power and minimize human errors. Ease of maintenance for these instruments is another important advantage of MFL comparing with other methods required heavy instrumentation.

The advanced MFL with optimized reaction systems and semi-automated procedures is expected to be a reliable and practical method for population based-multiple screening of the newborn metabolic diseases.

References

1. Guthrie R, Susi A. A simple phenylalanine method for detecting phenylketonuria in large populations of newborn infants. Pediatrics 1963;32:338–43.
2. Paigen K, Pacholec F, Levy HL. A new method of screening for inherited disorders of galactose metabolism. J Lab Clin Med 1982;99:895–907.
3. Hoffman GL, Laessig RH, Hassemer DJ, et al. Dual-channel continuous-flow system for determination of phenylalanine and galactose: application to newborn screening. Clin Chem 1984;30:287–90.
4. Rudy JL, Rutledge JC, Lewis SL. Phenylalanine and tyrosine in serum and eluates from dried blood spots as determined by reversed-phase liquid chromatography. C Lin Chem 1987;33:152–4.
5. Chance DH, Millington DS. New horizons in neonatal screening. Amsterdam: Excerpta Medica, 1994.
6. Yamaguchi A, Fukushi M, Mizushima Y, et al. Microassay for screening newborns for galactosemia with use of a fluorometric microplate reader. Clin Chem 1989;35:1962–4.
7. Gerasimova NS, Samutin AA, Steklova IV and Tuuminen T, et al.

Phenylketonuria screening in Moscow using a microplate fluorometric method. Screening 1992;1:27–35.

8. Yamaguchi A, Mizushima Y, Fukushi M, et al. Microassay system for newborn screening for phenylketonuria, maple syrup urine disease, homocystinuria, histidinemia and galactosemia with use of a fluorometric microplate reader. Screening 1992;1:49–62.

9. Yamaguchi A, Fukushi M, Sato Y, et al. Advanced microfluorometry for newborn screening for galactosemia and maple syrup urine disease. (under submission)

10. Yamaguchi A, Fukushi M, Sato Y, et al. Advanced microfluorometry for newborn homocystinuria screening. (under submission)

Tests for the Medium-chain Acyl-CoA Dehydrogenase (MCAD) Mutations, A985G and G583A, in Infants who Died from Sudden Infant Death Syndrome (SIDS)

H Mountain[1], A Ryan[2], J McGill[3], I Francis[3]*

[1] *Molecular Genetics Laboratory, Royal Brisbane Hospital, Brisbane, Australia.*
[2] *Department of Human Genetics, University of Newcastle-upon-Tyne, Newcastle, U.K.* [3] *Victorian Clinical Genetics Services, The Murdoch Institute, Melbourne, Australia.* ** Corresponding author.*

Abstract *Disorders of fatty acid oxidation have been shown to cause sudden death in infancy, and have an association with SIDS. We investigated the frequency of MCAD deficiency in a population of infants who had died of SIDS using assays for the A985G and G583A mutations. Dried blood spot samples from infants who had died suddenly without a definitive diagnosis (SIDS) were analyzed for 2 mutations of the MCAD gene. A985G is the most common mutation in Caucasians with MCAD deficiency, and has a frequency of 90% in mutant alleles. This suggests that 80% of cases are homozygous for this mutation. G583A is associated with a severe MCAD deficiency, and may be present in 1–2% of mutant alleles. 7 infants were found to be heterozygous for the A985G mutation. No infants had the G583A mutation. MCAD deficiency in infants homozygous for A985G was not a major cause of SIDS in this population, though this approach may miss some cases. Mass spectrometry for MCAD deficiency in a newborn population has shown a higher incidence than expected (1/8,930 as opposed to 1/13,000), and less than half were homozygous for A985G. This suggests that MCAD is under-diagnosed.*

Introduction

MCAD deficiency is an autosomal recessive disorder, which blocks the β-oxidation of 6–14 carbon unit fatty acids. It is characterized by periodic crises of hypoketotic hypoglycaemia, resembling 'Reye syndrome', which are precipitated by periods of fasting. MCAD deficiency can present with life-threatening symptoms in the neonatal period[1,2], and has been suggested as the cause of death in 1.5–5% of infants diagnosed as SIDS[3].

In Caucasian communities, the A985G mutation occurs at a frequency of 90% in cases of MCAD deficiency[4]. The expected birth incidence of A985G homozygotes, based on the population frequency of the A985G mutation[5], is 1/13,000 to 1/20,000. A second mutation, G583A, has been associated with severe MCAD deficiency and sudden infant death, and is thought to occur in 1–2% of mutant alleles. In order to determine the contribution of MCAD deficiency to SIDS in the Australian population, we have analyzed dried blood spot samples from 708 infants who died of SIDS for the 2 mutations, A985G and G583A.

Methods

Dried blood spot samples   Autopsy records for the years 1982–1990 were scanned for infants who had died suddenly without a definitive diagnosis (SIDS). 414 infants born in Victoria, and 294 infants born in Queensland were identified, and their dried blood spot specimens retrieved from storage for mutation analysis.

The A985G mutation   All 708 cards were analyzed by the method of Matsubara et al. PCR was performed using his primers 2 and 3; where primer 3 is mismatched and introduces an Nco 1 recognition site, CCATGG, in the mutated sequence.

The forward primer with normal and mutated sequences is:

```
                                              mismatch↓
primer 3F                5′ TGCTGGCTGAAATGGCCATG 3′
normal sequence .......    TGCTGGCTGAAATGGCAATGAaagttgaacta ....
mutated sequence ......     TGCTGGCTGAAATGGCAATGGaagttgaacta ....
                                              mutation↑
```

The reverse primer is:

```
primer 2R                3′ AATGGTCTCTCGTCGAACCC 5′
```

The PCR product is 63 bp. Dot blot hybridization was carried out with a digoxigenin labelled normal probe (5′ dTGGCCATGAAAGTTGAA 3′) and a mutant probe (5′ dTTCAACTTCCATGGCCA 3′). Confirmation of the dot blot findings was performed for the 294 Queensland samples by

Nco I digestion followed by gel electrophoresis. The normal sequence gives a 63 bp fragment and the mutated sequence gives a 43 bp fragment

The G583A mutation The 414 cards from Victoria were analyzed for this mutation. PCR was performed using a mismatched primer to introduce an Msp 1 recognition site, CCGG, in the normal sequence.

The forward primer with normal and mutated sequences is:

mismatch↓

primer 9F	5′ tggtcagaagatgtgggataacca<u>C</u>c 3′
normal sequence	tggtcagaagatgtgggataaccaacggaggaa ....
mutated sequence	tggtcagaagatgtgggataaccaac<u>A</u>gaggaa ....

mutation↑

The reverse primer is:

primer 8R	3′ GTCAATTCCATACAAACACCTTAAGCTTCC 5′

The normal and mutated amplified sequences were differentiated by Msp 1 digestion followed by gel electrophoresis. The normal sequence gives a 147 bp fragment and the mutated sequence gives a 172 bp fragment

Results

No infants homozygous for the A985G mutation were identified in the 708 infants tested. 7 infants (1 from Victoria and 6 from Queensland) were heterozygous for the mutation. The frequency of the mutation found in the SIDS infants (1/101) is at the low end of that expected in the general population (1/44 to 1/106). Of the known MCAD deficient patients, all 6 from Queensland, and 7 of 8 from Victoria, are homozygous for A985G. The other Victorian is heterozygous.

None of the infants tested (all from Victoria) had the G583A mutation.

Discussion

The failure to find cases of MCAD deficiency which is homozygous for the A985G mutation, agrees with other retrospective investigations into the association between MCAD deficiency and SIDS[6,7]. In these investigations, as in ours, the frequency of the A985G mutation did not differ significantly from that found in the general population. The selection of infants for this study was based upon the diagnosis of SIDS as the cause of death in the autopsy report. This selective process might have excluded some cases where pre-existing symptoms were suggestive of MCAD deficiency, but did not meet the diagnosis of SIDS.

Ziadeh et al.[8], using tandem mass spectrometry, detected 9 cases of MCAD deficiency from a prospective study of 80,371 newborns at a frequency of 1/8,930. A985G homozygotes accounted for only 4 of these cases, the remainder were A985G compound heterozygotes. This suggests that MCAD deficiency is more prevalent than previously thought, and that reliance on A985G homozygosity will miss many cases. MCAD deficiency is underdiagnosed in Victoria and Queensland. Diagnosis of unrelated cases relies upon metabolic studies after the onset of symptoms. There are 14 known cases, when, by A985G frequency alone, there should be at least 7 new cases each year.

The high frequency of the disorder in Caucasians, the early onset of severe symptoms, its association with infant mortality, its apparent under-diagnosis, and the availability of simple and effective dietary treatment, suggests it as a candidate for neonatal screening of selected populations. More studies are required to determine whether the missing cases are all asymptomatic, or include undiagnosed cases of neonatal death.

References

1. Brackett JC, Sims HF, Steiner RD, et al. A novel mutation in medium-chain acyl-CoA dehydrogenase causes sudden neonatal death. J Clin Invest 1994;94:1477–83.

2. Wilcken B, Carpenter KH and Hammond J. Neonatal symptoms in medium-chain acyl coenzyme A dehydrogenase deficiency. Arch Dis Child 1993; 69:292–4.

3. Bennett MJ, Allison F, Pollit RJ, Variend S. Fatty acid oxidation defects as causes of unexpected death in infancy. In: Tanaka K and Coates P, ed. Fatty acid oxidation: clinical biochemical and molecular aspects. New York: Alan R Liss, Inc, 1990:349–64.

4. Matsubara Y, Narisawa K, Tada K, et al. Identification of a common mutation in patients with medium-chain acyl-CoA dehydrogenase deficiency. Biochem Biophys Res Comm 1990;171:498–505.

5. Matsubara Y, Narisawa K, Tada K, et al. Prevalence of K329E mutation in medium-chain acyl-CoA dehydrogenase gene determined from Guthrie cards. Lancet 1991;338:552–3.

6. Miller ME, Brooks JG, Forbes N, Insel R. Frequency of medium-chain acyl-CoA deficiency G985 mutation in sudden infant death syndrome. Pediatr Res 1992;31:305–7.

7. Lundemose JB, Gregersen N, Klvraa S, et al. The frequency of a disease-causing point mutation in the gene coding for medium-chain acyl-CoA dehydrogenase in sudden infant death syndrome. Acta Paediatr 1993;82: 544–6.

8. Ziadeh R, Hoffman EP, Finegold DN, et al. Medium-chain acyl-CoA dehydrogenase deficiency in Pennsylvania: neonatal screening shows high incidence and unexpected mutation frequencies. Pediatr Res 1995;37:675–8.

Non-invasive Prenatal Diagnosis by Isolation of Both Trophoblasts and Foetal Nucleated Red Blood Cells from the Peripheral Blood of Pregnant Women

DTY Liu*, LG Durrant, KM McDowell, RA Holmes

*Academic Department of Clinical Oncology and Obstetrics, City Hospital, Nottingham, England. * Corresponding author.*

Abstract *Both trophoblast and fetal nucleated red cells are present in the peripheral circulation of pregnant women. Although few in numbers these cells can be isolated and with modern molecular genetic techniques will provide a definitive diagnosis. This is a major advantage over biochemical screening which at best offers a prediction. Protagonist for use of fetal cells as a screening technique favour either nucleated red cells or trophoblast. Our preliminary study showed recruitment of fetal cells in maternal blood is improved when both trophoblast and nucleated red cells are isolated simultaneously. When we applied our own monoclonal antibody (340) and anti-transferrin to the same maternal blood sample to sort fetal cells by PCR of the Y chromosome, correct sex was predicted in 83% (12 out of 13) of cases. Of importance is that the techniques were complimentary. No false positive were diagnosed with either technique.*

There is current interest in introducing population screening of trisomy 21 for all expectant mothers. The biochemical analytes HCG and serum alpha foetal protein (SAFP) in maternal blood are most commonly examined at 16 gestational weeks for this purpose. Overlap in results between normal and abnormal together with the question of centiles in any biochemical test meant that this approach in screening cannot be comprehensive. Whatever cut off level is selected for indication of risk for trisomy 21 some 20 to 30% of affected foetuses will be missed.

Amniocentesis performed for those assigned as at risk can result in the loss of nearly as many normal foetuses as abnormal ones in the young pregnant population. A further caveat rest with late diagnosis and the unwelcomed trauma if discontinuation of pregnancy is an option.

There is good evidence of foetal cell traffic into the maternal circulation during pregnancy. Lymphocytes, nucleated red blood cell and trophoblast can escape into the blood and be harvested through venipuncture. Only small numbers are present, usually in the region of one cell per millilitre of maternal blood. The current challenge for the scientists is to develop a reliable method to isolate these cells. Once these cells are captured, application of contemporary molecular biological techniques such as PCR and FISH can potentially provide a safe approach to prenatal diagnosis. A definitive diagnosis will obviate the roulette of uncertainty proposed by use of biochemical analyte screening[1].

Lymphocytes are not useful. Expression of HLA antigens suggests ready elimination from the maternal circulation. There is suspicion that they may persist between pregnancies hence an inherent risk of false diagnosis. NRBC can also be eliminated because of incompatibility with the ABO antigens. Furthermore, pregnancy may encourage a baseline level of nucleated cells from the mother. Despite this reservations some cells are present to encourage exploitation for prenatal diagnosis.

Trophoblasts are embolized into the maternal circulation throughout pregnancy. There is theoretical support for their presence in the first trimester at a time when cells from the foetal circulation may not gain assess to the maternal blood compartment. The last decade saw many attempts to develop antibodies to isolate trophoblasts. Our approach differed in exploitation of the commonality between cancer and trophoblastic tissue. This approach led to identification of a monoclonal antibody to sarcoma which also has a high affinity for trophoblast.

The paucity of foetal cells in maternal circulation led to the logical deduction that there is value in utilizing all available cells for diagnosis. To test this concept we combined use of our antibody (Mab340) and a commercially available monoclonal; antibody CD71, to isolate trophoblast and NRBC from the same maternal venous sample. Magnetic beads coated with these monoclonal antibodies were used as the vehicle to extract the targeted foetal cells.

Our pilot study has shown it is possible to identify correctly foetal sex in more than 80% of maternal blood samples tested[2]. There is evidence that isolation of trophoblast and NRBC are complementary approaches —

further support that the principal is correct. For non-invasive prenatal diagnosis we have found isolation of both trophoblast and nucleated red blood cells holds merit and we feel this should be the recommended approach.

References

1. Adinolfi M. Non or minimally invasive prenatal diagnostic test on maternal blood samples or transcervical cells. Prenatal Diagnosis 1995;15:889–96.
2. Durrant LG, McDowell KM, Holmes RA and Liu DTY. Screening of monoclonal antibodies recognising oncofoetal antigens for isolation of trophoblast from maternal blood for prenatal diagnosis. Prenatal Diagnosis 1994;14:131–40.

Prospects

Future Prospects of Neonatal Screening in the Asian Pacific Area

Calvin CP Pang

Department of Chemical Pathology, Chinese University of Hong Kong, Shatin, Hong Kong.

Abstract *In the Asian Pacific area neonatal screening programmes for important congenital diseases are well established in some regions but not so in others. Although the large geographical area and vast ethnic diversity attribute to variation in frequencies of congenital diseases in different regions, some diseases are commonly found in many regions. Examples are the thalassaemias, congenital hypothyroidism (CH) and glucose-6-phosphate dehydrogenase (G6PD) deficiency. In future it can be envisaged that vision of medical scientists and support from governments will bring forth knowledge of frequencies of congenital diseases in regions where they are yet to be determined. More attention will be paid to neonatal screening of infectious diseases. Advanced technology involving sophisticated instrumentation will be used in more and more regions, where there will also be novel innovations of technique advances. There will also be more international links on exchange of technical knowhows and organizational skills. All these efforts will contribute to a better understanding of the occurrence, pathophysiology and genetics of congenital diseases, and consequently, be of benefits to their treatment, prevention and genetic counselling.*

Introduction

Early diagnosis can prevent the permanent damage of some preventable and treatable diseases. To screen for a certain disease in infants during the neonatal period requires the detection method to be easy, reliable, cost-effective and acceptable to the population. To justify a neonatal screening programme in a population for any congenital disease, there must be available treatment to enable a large number of potentially affected people to be restored to normal life. There is also the financial consideration. The cost of treatment, most probably institutionalizing, for the resulting cases of handicap if no neonatal screening, should be higher than the screening cost. In the Asian Pacific area some congenital and treatable diseases do occur at high frequencies and demand neonatal screening.

In some regions such neonatal screening programmes are well in place. Examples are glucose-6-phosphate dehydrogenase deficiency and congenital hypothyroidism in regions like Japan, Taiwan, Singapore and Hong Kong. There are ethnic and regional differences in the occurrence of congenital diseases. In Japan a nationwide neonatal study was carried out between 1977 and 1982. A total of 6,311,754 newborns were investigated, coverage rate 87.7%[1]. The incidence of phenylketonuria (PKU) was found to be 1/109,000. Among the Chinese, regional screening programmes for PKU in different sites have revealed an incidence of 1/16,500 in Beijing, 1/17,000 in Shanghai and 1/33,000 in Taiwan[2,3,4]. These incidence rates are similar to the Caucasians but higher than the Japanese. In Hong Kong, where the population is predominantly Chinese originated from southern China, no case of PKU has been documented[5] and the incidence is highly likely to be very low[6]. Such a strong regional difference in PKU among the Chinese is striking.

A lot more about congenital diseases are still to be investigated, especially in regions where the incidence rates are yet to be determined. Sophisticated technology should be applied for rapid and accurate detection and for in-depth study on the transmission and genetics of prevalent congenital diseases. Meanwhile, neonatal screening for some infectious diseases does demand more attention in different regions.

Frequencies of specific congenital diseases

Knowledge of the frequencies of a congenital disease in a region is prerequisite for any consideration of neonatal screening. Such information is still unavailable in many regions in the Asian Pacific area even though occurrence of many congenital diseases have been reported. This can only be achieved by large-scale neonatal screening programmes. Diseases known to exist in high frequencies in the area should be investigated in all regions, notable examples being PKU, G6PD deficiency and congenital hypothyroidism (CHT). There are reliable and established methodology for the detection of these diseases. Meanwhile, dried blood spots on Guthrie paper provide an extremely effective and reliable method of blood sampling. Blood collection is easy because only blood spots, usually by heel prick, are required. Transport of such samples is not difficult even in remote areas or in regions not with efficient transport system. No stringent conditions for transport are required and they can be sent by post or courier.

Certainly in some populations there are congenital diseases with high frequencies. Many are yet to be discovered. Large population screening have to be carried out in many regions. Knowledge of disease patterns is important for health care in a population. It also provides a foundation for detailed investigation to advance our understanding of population genetics, molecular genetics and transmission of diseases. Population screening should also be extended for the detection of genetic susceptibility to disease, particularly common and severe diseases such as cancers and cardiovascular diseases[7].

New Technology

There are established methods of detection for many congenital diseases, such as the detection of hyperphenylalaninaemia by chromatographic analysis or by the Guthrie test. Continuous efforts are still needed for the advancement of techniques for cost-effective and reliable diagnosis. Such methods also have to be easy to be suitable for use for large-scale screening. Advances in automated analyzers for immunoassays are important but methods utilizing this approach have to be inexpensive to be useful in regions not economically effluent.

Bioanalytical mass spectrometry provides reliable information-rich detection of metabolites in body fluids for the identification of inherited metabolic diseases. Gas chromatography-mass fragmentography (GCMS) utilizing high resolution capillary GC columns and mass selective detectors is a well established method of profiling urinary organic acids for the detection of disorders in amino acid and organic acid metabolism[8,9]. Electron ionization on bench-top quadrupole mass spectrometers is adequate and reliable for total ion or selected ion analysis[10]. Advances in computer engineering and availability of effective and highly efficient derivatization reagents, notable example being bis-trimethyl-silyltrifluoroacetamide (BSTFA), have rendered GCMS to be an excellent method for larger-scale population screening.

Bioanalytical Mass Spectrometry Tandem mass spectrometry has also been applied to screening. Electrospray tandem mass spectrometry (ESI-MS/MS) can be fully automated for injection and MS analysis of sample molecules extracted from dried blood spots[11]. Quantitative measurements have been provided for homocystine, methionine, acylcarnitine, methyl-malonic acid and other amino and organic acid residues[11,12,13]. No chemical derivatization is required in some protocols. Tandem mass spectrometry is much more sensitive, specific, rapid and versatile than GCMS. It is much more powerful in mass ionization and is capable to analyze non-volatile or thermally unstable compounds even if they exist in ion forms in solution. Modern tandem quadrupole mass spectrometer and computerization provides rapid analysis and data interpretation. The main disadvantage of tandem mass spectrometer is its cost, not just the capital equipment cost but also supporting facilities including ventilation and maintenance. Specially trained technical personnel is needed. In regions where these are affordable, tandem MS would certainly be applied more and more for neonatal screening[14].

Molecular Techniques   The advent of polymerase chain reaction (PCR) has provided a powerful method for detection of DNA mutations leading to clinical phenotypes. For congenital diseases having known gene defects rapid and reliable protocols using recombinant DNA can be established for direct DNA diagnosis. One notable example is cystic fibrosis in which the 3-base pair deletion leading to a loss in phenylalanine in codon 508 of the cystic fibrosis gene (cystic fibrosis transmembrane conductance regulator, CFTR) accounts for as many as 75% of Caucasian CF patients[15]. Short deletions of the dystrophin gene occurs in about 60% of Duchenne Muscular Dystrophy[16] and the expansion of CGG trinucleotide repeats in the FMR-1 gene is the cause of the Fragile X syndrome of mental retardation[17]. Direct DNA diagnostic methods are available for these diseases and they can be applied for neonatal screening. In diseases with heterogeneous mutations in the candidate gene screening methods are available to detect base changes. One of the most popular method is single strand conformation polymorphism (SSCP) which utilizes native polyacrylamide electrophoresis of PCR products for detection of base changes. Using the PCR-SSCP methodology, possible common mutations have been detected in the low density lipoprotein receptor gene in Chinese familial hypercholesterolaemia patients in Hong Kong[18]. Identification of specific mutations also provides the basis to study the pattern of inheritance and penetrance of gene mutations in a population. Meanwhile, gene study is necessary to screen for susceptibility of diseases[7]. It is anticipated that more protocols of direct DNA analysis will be established to be suitable for neonatal screening and for genetic investigations.

Screening for Infectious Diseases

There are more and more concern on non-genetic diseases such as infectious diseases which lead to increased risk of intrauterine infections. The high incidence of hepatitis in many regions in Asia and the vertical transmission of the hepatitis B virus have led to the establishment of neonatal screening and vaccination programmes in some countries. The high frequency of HIV infections in some regions is alarming. The risk of HIV transmission from an infected mother to the fetus may be as high as 40%[19] based on studies in the United States. Highly effective screening programmes are in need to detect infected women of child-bearing age and newborn carriers. Rapid, reliable and cost-effective methods of detection have to be established and screening programmes have to be well organized.

New International Links

The Asian Pacific area is not only characterized by diversity in culture and ethnicity but also wide variation in the development of screening programmes. Some regions are advanced in technical knowhows and rich in organizational experiences. In these regions there will be continuous progress in application of new technology for in-depth research and wide population study of congenital diseases. In many others regions even the frequencies of common congenital diseases are not known. There are also regions, usually in more remote areas, where consangeous marriages are common and are therefore more prone to clustering of genetic diseases. Exchanges and collaboration among the international community will help regions needing technical knowhows and organizational experiences. More about congenital diseases will also be discovered and more detailed investigations should be carried out in regions where such studies are lacking. The First Asian Pacific Regional Meeting of the International Society of Neonatal Screening held at Sapporo, Japan in 1993 was instrumental to bring in workers in the Asian Pacific area to discuss about neonatal screening for the first time. The success of the first meeting led to good attendance and wide coverage of topics in the second meeting in Hong Kong in 1995. It is anticipated that in the third meeting in Thailand there will be even larger attendance, more complete representation from all regions in the Asian Pacific area and more reports of screening programmes being out carried out in different regions. International meetings of such are extremely helpful for exchange of knowledge and experiences and for establishment of contacts for collaboration. Meanwhile, there should also be more international exchange of visits of workers in neonatal screening. Experienced and established workers should have the opportunity to share their expertise with workers in regions having less development of screening programmes.

Conclusion

Apart from vision and devotions of workers in medical genetics financial support is the major need for any study on congenital diseases. Very often funding has to be provided by the state. The world's fastest growing economies are now mostly found in the Asian Pacific area. Hopefully economic growth would enable more government support for the study of congenital diseases.

References

1. Tada K, Tateda H, Arashima S, et al. Follow-up study of a nation-wide neonatal metabolic screening promgram in Japan. Eur J Pediatr 1984; 142:204–7.
2. Liu SR, Zuo QH. Newborn screening for phenylketonuria in eleven districts. Chin Med J 1986;99:113–8.
3. Chen RG, Pan XS, Qian DL, Guo H. Twenty-one cases of phenylketonuria out of 358,767 newborns in Shanghai, China. J Inher Metab Dis 1989;12:485.
4. Hsiao KJ. Genetic disorders and neonatal screening. In: Miyai K, Kanno T, Ishikawa E, ed. Progress in clinical biochemistry. New York: Elsevier Science Publishers, 1992:289–92.
5. Davies DP. Paediatric illness ion Hong Kong and Britain. Arch Dis Child 1992;67:543–9.
6. Pang CCP, Chan AKH, Poon PMK, et al. Inborn errors of metabolism in children with mental retardation. HK J Paediatr 1994;11:133–8.
7. Clarke A. Population screening for genetic susceptibility to disease. Brit Med J 1995;311:35–8.
8. Lefevere MF, Verhaeghe BJ, Declerch DM, De Leenheer AP. Asutomated profiling of urinary organic acids by dual-column gas chromatograpghy and gas chromatography/mass spectrometry. Biomed Environ Mass spect 1988; 15:311–22.
9. Shih VE. Detection of hereditary metabolic disorders involving amino acids and organic acids. Clin Biochem 1991;24:301–9.

10. Pang CCP. Laboratory investigation of inherited metabolic diseases. HK Med J 1996 (in press).

11. Rashed MS, Ozand PT, Bucknall MP, Little D. Diagnosis of inborn errors of metabolism from blood spots by acylcarnitines and amino acids profiling using automated electrospray tandem mass spectrometry. Pediatr Res 1995; 38:324–31.

12. Chace DH, Hillman SL, Millington DS, et al. Rapid diagnosis of homocyctinuria and other hypermethioninemias from newborn's blood spots by tandem mass spectrometry. Clin Chem 1996;42:349–55.

13. Rashed MS, Ozand PT, Harrison ME, et al. Electrospray tandem mass spectrometry in the diagnosis of organic acidemias. Rapid Comm Mass Spect 1994;8:129–33.

14. Millington DS, Terada N, Kodo N, Chace DH. A review: carnitine and acylcarnitine analysis in the diagnosis of metabolic diseases. Advantages of tandem mass spectrometry. In: Matsumoto I, ed. Advance in chemical diagnosis and treatment of metabolic disorders, Vol I. New York: Wiley, 1992:59–71.

15. The Cystic Fibrosis Genetic Analysis Consortium. Worldwide survey of the delta F508 mutation: report from the Cystic Fibrosis Genetic Analysis Consortium. Am J Hum Genet 1990;47:354.

16. Abbs S, Bobrow M. Analysis of quantitative PCR for the diagnosis of deletion and duplication carriers in the dystrophin gene. J Med Genet 1992;29:191–6.

17. Fu YH, Kuhl DPA, Pizzuti A, et al. Variation of the CGG repeat at the Fragile X site results in genetic instability: resolutuion of the Sherman Paradox. Cell 1991;67:1047–58.

18. Mak YT, Zhang J, Chan YS, et al. Possible common mutation in the low density lipoprotein receptor gene in Chinese. Hum Mutat 1996 (in press).

19. Davis SF, Byers RH, Lindegren ML, et al. Prevalence and incidence of vertically acquired HIV infection in the United States. JAMA 1995;247:952–5.

Issues in Implementation of Neonatal and Perinatal Screening Programmes

Stephen TS Lam

Clinical Genetic Service, Department of Health, Cheung Sha Wan Jockey Club Clinic, Shamshuipo, Hong Kong.

Abstract *With advances in technology and increasing emphasis for preventive care, screening programmes for genetic and non-genetic disorders have received increasing attention in the past few decades. In the following article, some issues of significance in the implementation of these programmes are discussed. These issues involve health care policy, funding, socio-ethical considerations and quality assurance.*

For the past three decades, neonatal screening for inherited metabolic diseases and endocrinopathies have been well established in preventive and public health medicine in many regions in the world. This was the result of two major lines of development. To start with, developments in technologies have allowed for better means of sampling, transporting and storing human specimens; more sensitive and specific methods of analysis of metabolites, proteins, and genes to detect abnormalities; and more powerful ways of collating and transmitting information by the computer technology. In addition, it is gradually realized that the future emphasis of health care should be on preventive care and public health medicine. More governments are now convinced of the significant role of screening for congenital disorders as a secondary measure of prevention, and policies are devised and implemented accordingly. During the past years, the spectrum of diseases screened during the neonatal period has been extended to include other genetic disorders and congenital infections.

For these screening programmes to be successfully implemented, developments in technology must be complemented by the appropriate health policy. In this regard, four specific issues should be considered.

Firstly, in the realm of public health and preventive medicine, the primary aim is to safeguard the health of the whole population via the provision of a efficient and effective health care services. This has to be directed by a health policy developed appropriately for that population. The questions to be asked are: 'What diseases should be screened?'; 'Which should come first?'; 'What are the social or political implications?'. It should be realized that the answer to these questions can change with time, hence the constant changes in priorities. For example, a disease without known treatment may not be considered for inclusion in a screening programme. However, as technology advances, treatment may become a reality in some diseases which were regarded as untreatable, and the issue needs to be reconsidered. Duchenne muscular dystrophy offers a good illustration[1] and more and more examples are expected in future.

The second issue concerns financing screening programmes. Given that an individual programme receives health policy support, there still remains the major question of 'who to pay?' In Hong Kong, neonatal screening for some conditions are considered priorities by the government. These are publicly funded and are provided universally to all newborns in Hong Kong[2,3]. However, funding mechanisms are found to be different in various countries[4], because of differences in their economic structure and social policy. Every country has to take these factors into consideration before implementation of any screening programme.

Thirdly, population screening is fraught with arguments on rights of the individuals. The issues of confidentiality, informed consent, perception of burden to individuals and the society, autonomy of individuals in making choices and the right to use left over specimens for alternative purposes are often brought to public debate. Some countries tend to be more 'directive' than can be tolerated in another. This necessarily submit any screening endeavours to social, cultural and political scrutiny.

Finally, all screening programmes and systems need to be properly managed. Part of their management concerns quality assurance (QA). While internal QA efforts have be built in as an integral part of most screening system, more emphasis should now be given to external QA, since this can further safeguard the integrity and quality of the programmes. It is hence important to establish and maintain international networks of collaboration. More international efforts and collaboration are required.

References

1.   Bradley DM, Parsons EP, Clarke A. Preliminary experience with newborn screening for Duchenne muscular dystrophy. Brit Med J 1993; 360:357–60.

2. Lo KK, Chan ML, Lo IFM, Lai SSL, Li KCK, Hung P, Lam STS. Neonatal screening for glucose-6-phosphate dehydrogenase deficiency in Hong Kong. This book:33.
3. Lo KK, Lam STS. Neonatal screening programme for congenital hypothyroidism in Hong Kong. This book:145.
4. Takasugi N and Naruse J. New trends in neonatal screening. Sapporo: Hokkaido University Press, 1994.

Index